PRAISE FOR DANIELLE HAWKINS

When It All Went to Custard

'An emotional rollercoaster ride, with a fair serve of humour and heart'

'Funny, hopeful and big-hearted, *When It All Went to Custard* is a story about family, farming, second chances, and finding your feet. Fans of Marian Keyes, Sophie Kinsella and Cecelia Ahern are guaranteed to love it' Better Reading

'The special treat in store is the witty dialogue, and especially the way Hawkins captures the offbeat things kids say and do, and the insight into small-community, country life' Stuff NZ

The Pretty Delicious Café

'Everything a summer read should be … Warm and witty' *Who Weekly*

'*The Pretty Delicious Café* is brimming with romance and eccentricity. A refreshing take on romantic comedy, it reminds us about the importance of family, friends and the opportunity of fresh beginnings' Better Reading

'… hits the mark with its quaint and cosy setting, smattering of eccentric small-town characters and budding romance' *Weekly Times*, Melbourne

'*The Pretty Delicious Café* is another delightful read from Danielle Hawkins. It's light-hearted, self-deprecating and charming, with quirky and engaging characters' *The Blurb* magazine

'*Pretty Delicious* is a story of determination, of love, of allowing oneself the freedom to follow their dreams … It is a story of friendship … and the power of reconciliation and forgiveness. The characters, with their flaws and neuroses are heartbreakingly real, and thus easy to identify with' The Bookseller New Zealand blog

'I loved this book, I love the characters and I love the sense of family' Beauty & Lace Book Club pick

'Danielle Hawkins … has a talent for witty and convincing dialogue and this, in particular, gives *The Pretty Delicious Café* verve and humour. She's also a skilled sculptor of characters' *Otago Daily Times*

'Danielle Hawkins' quirky humour and easy style make this a great summer read' *Dominion Post*

'Delightful is a perfect description … it really is a wonderful story, with quirky and relatable characters, fast, witty dialogue and lots of humour' NicShef♥Reading #1 reviewer Amazon

Chocolate Cake for Breakfast

'Another sweet, gently funny depiction of life in the back blocks of New Zealand' *Next* Book Club

'This is a delightful, contemporary romance' *Herald Sun*

'Helen is frankly delightful – intelligent but oh-so-human … a plausible, relatable storyline and hugely appealing characters. A charming summer read, and a giggling good time' *Australian Women's Weekly*

'Helen reminds me of a modern day James Herriot and her often hilarious adventures in this dairy country will have you laughing (although if you're squeamish this may not be the book for you!)' Bec, GoodReads

'This is pure escapism and I thoroughly enjoyed this read' Carol, Reading Writing and Riesling

'This book is like chocolate cake for breakfast: addictive' Bree T, GoodReads

Dinner at Rose's

'It's so good that it's hard to believe it's a first novel. It had better not be her last. Please, Danielle' Lee Matthews, *Manawatu Standard*

'What really carries it is the quality of the writing. The dialogue is absolutely spot on. You would almost believe the author wrote for TV or writes sitcoms. It's very, very funny' Paper Plus, Winter Reads

'A cross between *All Creatures Great and Small*, *Bridget Jones's Diary* and something the Topp Twins would write if there was only one of them and she was straight, this is a very funny book' *Next* Book Club

'It was page 4 when I saw this and knew it was going to be a good book: "You really should consider becoming an eccentric yourself. It makes life so much more interesting"' Jessica, GoodReads

'I LOVED this book and devoured it quickly' Georgia, GoodReads

'This book … has to be the most satisfying in this genre that I've ever read' Kathleen Dixon, GoodReads

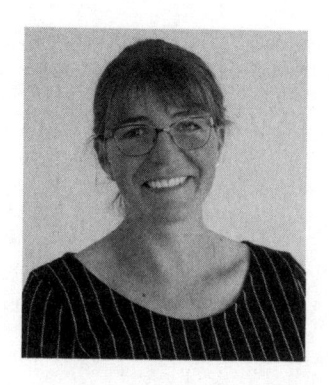

Danielle Hawkins lives on a sheep and beef farm near Otorohanga in New Zealand with her husband and two children, and works part-time as a vet. She is a keen gardener and conservationist, and an expert French-plaiter. She can be found on Facebook at @DanielleHawkinsAuthor, where she posts seldom and grudgingly but is good at replying to messages.

Also by Danielle Hawkins

Dinner at Rose's
Chocolate Cake for Breakfast
The Pretty Delicious Café
When It All Went to Custard

TWO SHAKES OF A LAMB'S TAIL

The Diary of a Country Vet

TWO SHAKES OF A LAMB'S TAIL

The Diary of a Country Vet

Danielle Hawkins

HarperCollinsPublishers

HarperCollinsPublishers
Australia • Brazil • Canada • France • Germany • Holland • Hungary
India • Italy • Japan • Mexico • New Zealand • Poland • Spain • Sweden
Switzerland • United Kingdom • United States of America

First published in 2021
by HarperCollins*Publishers* (New Zealand) Limited
Unit D1, 63 Apollo Drive, Rosedale, Auckland 0632, New Zealand
harpercollins.co.nz

Copyright © Danielle Hawkins 2021

Danielle Hawkins asserts the moral right to be identified as the author of this work. This work is copyright. All rights reserved. No part of this publication may be reproduced, copied, scanned, stored in a retrieval system, recorded, or transmitted, in any form or by any means, without the prior written permission of the publisher.

A catalogue record for this book is available from the National Library of New Zealand.

ISBN 978 1 7755 4158 5 (pbk)
ISBN 978 1 7754 9189 7 (ebook)

Cover design by Darren Holt, HarperCollins Design Studio
Cover images: Wellington boots by Simon Belcher / Getty Images; Lambs by shutterstock.com
Poo emoji by shutterstock.com
Typeset in Baskerville Regular by Kirby Jones
Author photograph by Marama Shearer, Thrive Photography
Printed and bound in Australia by McPherson's Printing Group
The papers used by HarperCollins in the manufacture of this book are a natural, recyclable product made from wood grown in sustainable plantation forests. The fibre source and manufacturing processes meet recognised international environmental standards, and carry certification.

To Jarrod

*Sometimes I wonder how you put up with me,
and then I remember that I put up with you.*

Introduction

A year or so ago, I was trying to write a book combining the grandeur and originality of *Northern Lights* with the delicate charm of *Pride and Prejudice*, and it wasn't going all that well, when I got an email from my publisher suggesting I might like to try my hand at writing something true for a change: a book about rural life.

It sounded like fun, and a good excuse to put that frustrating, not-working novel to one side. So I started a diary, thinking that would give a nice overview of a typical farming year. The fact that 2020 ended up having a global pandemic in the middle of it made the year less typical than I was expecting, but such is life.

We – my husband, two children and I – live on a sheep farm halfway down the North Island. We farm 1200 ewes and 400 cattle, on 460 hectares of rolling hill country. Around three-quarters of the farm is in grass, the rest is native bush, and I think it's the nicest place in the world, although I know I'm biased.

I work part-time as a large-animal vet, help on the farm and write in my spare time. Because the spare time is fairly limited, the writing tends to be accompanied by guilt at not doing something more useful, like filling bait stations or spraying gorse.

This diary isn't *entirely* true, because I decided that faithfully reproducing my friends and relatives in print probably wasn't the best idea, but it's as accurate a record as I could write without hurting anyone's feelings or being accused of defamation of character.

Despite my low-level guilt at cutting into bait-station-filling time, I've had a lovely time writing this book. I hope you like it.

Danielle Hawkins

Monday 15 July

Maternal fashion at the school bus stop reached a new low this morning. I was wearing fluffy slippers, polar fleece trackpants (very unflattering) and a khaki-coloured polar fleece jumper. Amy, who lives just down the road, was in a grubby dressing-gown and gumboots, and Jaide from up the road was in shiny camo-patterned tights and an egg-stained hoodie. None of us had brushed our hair.

I am so grateful not to live in a smart suburb where the other mothers have expensive highlights and wear Lululemon.

Tuesday 16 July

The pet pigs are deeply unimpressed by the weather. It has rained without stopping for the last 30 hours, with one mini tornado by way of variation. We got home tonight to find them both camped in the carport, having found their way through two fences. They were soothed by half a pot of leftover soup (pea and ham, but what they don't know won't hurt them) and four Anzac biscuits.

Wednesday 17 July

It rained all night. I woke at intervals to worry about newborn lambs and fantails and other small, cute things that were out in it, and then fell deeply asleep at 6 a.m. only to be woken at 6.10 by the lady who monitors the vet clinic phones after hours calling me to a prolapse. While I got dressed, James made me two cups of coffee, bless him – one to drink on the way and the other in a thermos-cup for afterwards.

It was an enormous prolapse, and both it and the cow (who was down) were covered in mud. The paddock looked like the Somme. It was raining and only just light, but the couple who own the farm and their nice Filipino worker had never seen a prolapsed uterus before, and they were so excited that all three of them came to help.

It was marvellous. Normally with prolapses you cradle a great lump of swollen, red, inside-out uterus on your lap, trying to lift it and get it back in with the help of one assistant, who is usually small and feeble and wants to be somewhere else. But this time I had two cheerful, strapping men to lift the uterus, and a third assistant to keep it clean and covered in lube as I pushed and shoved and folded and massaged it back inside the cow where it belonged. That well-known stage of prolapse replacement, where you're exhausted and wondering why you ever thought that anyone would ever be able to thread a lump of tissue the size of a fat Labrador through a hole the size of a grapefruit, was bypassed entirely.

Thursday 18 July

Today I was supposed to spend the morning at home – it feels at the moment as if I'm never there, certainly not for long enough to do anything useful like housework or gardening – but no. James appeared back at the door ten minutes after he'd left, saying that

Dream, the heading dog, had just eaten the remains of a mouldy bag of possum bait off the rubbish fire pile at the woolshed. (My fault, as he explained at some length, for throwing mouldy possum bait into the bin when I got home from checking bait stations last week.) So I took Dream – and Taz, in case he'd eaten it too – to the clinic and gave them apomorphine to make them vomit. Dream, horrible little grub that she is, had apparently washed down her snack of mouldy bait with sheep poo. That dog has no class.

Back at home I paid the bills, reconciled last month's accounts and wrestled with the PAYE. I have not yet mastered Payday Filing, mostly due to not caring enough to learn how to do it properly, so am anticipating a nasty letter from Inland Revenue any time now. While looking at my credit card statement (always depressing) I saw a strange transaction. Supposedly I had spent $50 at Toolking somewhere in Massachusetts, USA. Oh, shit, I thought, and rang the bank hotline.

Bad mistake.

First, I got my name wrong when they asked for it (my credit card is still in my maiden name; I never got around to changing it). Then I failed the security questions. 'What was your work phone number when you opened this account?' It was about twenty years ago! How the hell would I know? 'What was your most recent credit card purchase?' No idea. Groceries? Ellie's new sneakers?

I had a long and dispiriting conversation with a girl who was evidently wondering whether I was a criminal or just a moron, which ended when I remembered that I had bought a pair of fancy secateurs from a tiny stall at the Fieldays last month.

The feeling of being a complete twerp was not alleviated by reading an article about myself in *Newsroom*. The nice young journalist who came for lunch a few weeks ago has quoted me at length, verbatim, and I sound like Lyn of Tawa after a hard night on the piss. Judging by my family's hysterical laughter at the picture topping the article, I look like it too.

I was cheered up over dinner, though, when Blake asked: 'What colour was Dad's hair when it was still alive?'

Friday 19 July

I've done a terrible thing. I assumed the woman I was standing next to at the edge of the netball courts this afternoon was pregnant, and she's not. We were talking about calving – she and her husband work on a dairy farm – and I looked meaningfully at her stomach and said, '*You'll* be busy this spring!' There was a puzzled sort of silence before she said quietly, 'No, I'm not pregnant, I'm just fat.' Awful. Just awful. I bet she went home and cried. And I *know* the rules. You never, ever ask a woman when the baby is due *unless you can actually see a baby coming out of her*. In which case the question is unnecessary.

Sunday 21 July

I've just been sent an email outlining some potential questions for an upcoming author panel. (Not quite sure why I thought going to an evening event on a work night in the middle of calving was a good idea, but never mind.) The event's chair, a professor of literature, writes that we authors have wonderfully diverse voices, and our divergences and juxtapositions will give the evening a lot of its energy and interest. We all write about the forces that imprison, frustrate and seek to control humanity, but our characters seek to find purpose, meaning, escape and transcendence in vastly different ways. So she's going to direct the conversation along those lines.

After spending some time trying to translate her email into plain English, I *think* it means: 'All of you write about stuff that happens, and how people cope with it.' Isn't every book, play or movie ever written, from Shakespeare to *Peter Rabbit*, about stuff that happens and how people – or rabbits – cope with it?

There seems to be a big difference (or perhaps a deep-seated and fundamentally dichotomous philosophical shift) between my opinion about what makes writing good and that of the literary world. I think that the very best writing is easy to read – the writer finds the words that convey exactly what she's trying to say as simply as possible, so that the reader is swept up and forgets he's reading at all. Literary experts, however, seem to believe that the best writing is dense and elliptical, leaving the reader feeling dazed, exhausted and, preferably, slightly inadequate. (Also, books that win literary awards must be miserable. I don't think I'm a great writer, but I resent the assumption that anyone who writes light-hearted romantic fiction *can't* be a great writer.)

Friday 2 August

Highly productive day today. James and I planted 55 poplar poles at the back of the farm, where there isn't enough shade for the stock. Poplar poles aren't the most beautiful specimen trees, but each one comes with its own little protective plastic sleeve, so they don't each need a personal eight-wire fence. This is an important consideration. A few autumns ago, we bought a whole lot of baby trees – beeches, pohutukawas, nyssas (they have the best autumn colouring ever), sugar maples (second-best autumn colouring), flowering chestnuts, etc. The farm will look so pretty in 300 years that they'll probably make it into a World Heritage site, but by the time James had built a proper fence around each newly planted tree he was feeling a little sour. (In theory I'm a firm advocate of girls being able to do pretty much anything boys do, but in practice I hope to reach the end of my life without ever learning to fence, shear or weld.)

Monday 5 August

We have two lambs in a box in the laundry and four outside in a pen on the lawn. We're going to try feeding them ad lib this year, after last year's experience of feeding forty of the little dears four times a day for months on end. You wouldn't resent the hours and hours it takes – or at least you'd resent it less – if the lambs turned out looking amazing, but they were smallish and a bit pot-bellied and generally pretty average.

Eleven-year-old Ellie has announced grandly that she will spend at least an hour every afternoon training her lamb, but she's going to start tomorrow.

Blake, who is eight, has made no such declaration. He has recently taken to responding to any request by drooping like a piece of wilted lettuce and saying dully, 'Yes, Mum.' A witness would automatically conclude that I am a heartless oppressor who has crushed all spirit and happiness from my child, and to make it even more annoying, he evidently feels that as long as he agrees to do whatever I've asked him to do with the appropriate level of servility, *he doesn't actually have to do it.*

I was on call last weekend – the very height of calving season and historically the busiest after-hours weekend of the year. My best friend Clare, who has spent the last ten years building up a successful small-animal practice and is now having an if-I-spend-another-twenty-years-cleaning-cats'-teeth-will-I-really-have-made-the-world-a-better-place crisis, came down from Auckland to calve cows with me. She spent the whole week leading up to it sending me excited text messages about gumboots and waterproof leggings.

Friday night. No calvings. Dined on hamburgers and chocolate peppermint slice, watched *The Secret Life of Walter Mitty* and enjoyed the calm before the storm.

Saturday morning. No calvings. We went into the clinic at 9 a.m. and graciously agreed – while waiting for calvings – to see a cat with blood in its urine. I acted as vet nurse while Clare administered subcutaneous fluids, antibiotics and pain relief and booked the cat in for blood testing on Monday. Great to see the small-animal expert in action.

Over the next two hours we saw another cat with urinary issues, an injured pig dog, a puppy with diarrhoea and a cat with an abscess. We went home for lunch then spent the afternoon weeding the garden, which I thought was great but wasn't the afternoon Clare had hoped for.

Our first cow call was at dinner time. We drove for an hour and a quarter to the back of beyond – through gorgeous countryside, had we been able to see it – to a heifer with a breech calving. On arrival we found the shed in complete darkness, which was disconcerting, but after a while the farmer wandered down and turned the lights on. The heifer was sitting down on the yard. Clare did the initial check, and was so enthused by her findings that she immediately lay down behind the cow and vanished up to the shoulder. In about ten minutes she'd calved it. We got the heifer up then drove an hour and a quarter home.

On Sunday morning we actually had two calvings in a row. The first one was down in the mud in the middle of a hailstorm (rotten calf, pulled it out inch by laborious inch, spiking holes in it with a knife to let out the gas as it came), the second one down in a race (upside-down calf with the head twisted around). Both farmers were miserable – the first because he had failed to put on his wet-weather gear before ferrying the vets to the side of the cow and then watching them calve it in a hailstorm; the second because his manager has decided, in the second week of calving, that he doesn't think the dairy industry is quite his cup of tea after all and has gone on stress leave.

Clare then headed back to Auckland early to beat the traffic. I'm not sure her weekend was a very good example of the life of a dairy vet, but it was lovely to see her.

Thursday 8 August

My sister-in-law Diane (James's brother Thomas's wife; they live two kilometres up the road on the men's grandparents' original farm and are slightly superior to us in every way) just rang to ask why her mother's cat might be pacing the hall and yowling all night. How should I know?

She told me that they started lambing last Tuesday and they've all but finished. They've only seen about five dead lambs (they have 2000 ewes), and every triplet-bearing ewe is feeding all three.

She also told me that she finally started my new book a few weeks ago, having borrowed it from James's mum – it would never occur to her to buy one – but, somehow, she just couldn't get into it. 'I passed it on to Nicky Jones at the medical centre,' she said. 'She actually quite liked your last one.'

I hung up the phone in the state of indignant wrath Diane so often induces in me, and realised that I'd just tipped a little heap of diced pumpkin in the pig bucket and tossed the peelings into my soup. Rage and cooking do not mix well.

Monday 12 August

A very nice farmer rang me at work today and asked me to come out on Wednesday and remove the warts from the penis of one of his sale bulls. Having managed to evade penile wart removal in nineteen years of veterinary practice, I asked Bill, who has been a vet for forty years and knows everything, for advice.

Apparently, it's easy. You simply massage the bull's prostate glands per rectum for two or five or ten minutes; the penis becomes erect, an assistant at the bull's side grabs it as it emerges and holds on for grim death (if they miss it you've got another ten minutes of prostatic massage), you inject a little bleb of local anaesthetic at the base of each wart and burn them off with the electrocautery machine. Dear God. It sounds like an absolutely brilliant way to get your head kicked in.

*

I left work a little early to go and have my makeup done for the author panel. I felt I needed a small confidence boost before spending an evening talking about writing in the company of a couple of award-winning literary authors.

Nicolette Goudge, makeup expert, beautician, pessimist and all-round legend, is one of my favourite people. She maintained a steady flow of lament while she worked. 'Your skin is so dry. You spend far too much time outside. And these red cheeks – have you considered laser treatment for your broken capillaries? This eyebrow is crooked ...' Finally she decided she could do no more, shrugged and handed me the mirror. And I was beautiful. Like myself, only much better. Hooray!

Despite my fears, the author panel was lots of fun. The chair was a giggly and delightful lady, and she must have got all that stuff about divergences and juxtapositions out of her system in her email, because she spoke perfectly clear English. The other authors were charming – the most literary of them told us that the theme of his work is Identity and spoke at some length about his cultural relevance, but was actually quite nice in spite of it. We went out for dinner after the panel – all in all a very pleasant contrast to normal life. Probably best not to do it too often, though; I might start talking about my cultural relevance. On second thoughts, that's very unlikely, living with James.

Tuesday 13 August

Mrs Johnson came into the clinic today. Again.

I saw her little dog about a month ago. It was old and lethargic, with chronic skin problems, and she was wondering sadly if it was time to Make the Decision.

I examined the dog from nose to tail, and all I found was inflamed skin and an ear infection.

'She has cancer too,' said Mrs Johnson.

'Really?'

'In her glands. The other vet told me there was nothing we could do.'

I couldn't find any record of the cancer diagnosis on the computer, but I said – several times, because she seemed pretty wedded to the cancer idea – that I thought the lymph nodes *were* a bit enlarged, but that might well just be because her skin was so irritated.

We segued, at that point, into a long discussion about greenlipped mussel extract, which she was giving the dog but which frankly she had her doubts about. Eventually we returned to the matter at hand, and I prescribed a week's antibiotics and then a check-up to see how things were going.

She cancelled the revisit. I rang her, and she said she was worried about the cost of all these trips to the vet, and since her little dog had cancer she thought she'd just keep her quietly at home while she seemed to have reasonable quality of life. I promised faithfully not to charge her a fortune, and she came in. Dog much improved on antibiotics. Lymph nodes normal size. Cancer cloud lifted. Ear still a bit hot – I prescribed another week of antibiotics and sent her on her way rejoicing.

Today Mrs Johnson was back, bearing an enormous rabbit that needed its nails clipped. I asked after her little dog.

'Well,' she said, 'it's amazing! You know those green-lipped mussel pills? They're *wonderful*. I'm telling everyone about them. They cured my little dog of cancer, you know!'

Hmm.

Wednesday 14 August

Survived bull penile wart removal, after spending most of last night picturing all the ways in which it might go wrong. Prostatic massage was unnecessary; the wart was as big as a grapefruit, stopping the penis from going back into the prepuce at all. Knocked the bull right down, thus removing the risk of being kicked in the head. Surgery gory but safe. Whew.

I have three deep-blue hyacinths coming up among the daffodils in the orchard. They were given to me a couple of years ago in a pot, and when they'd finished flowering, I planted them out, never expecting to see them again. And there they are, bless them, pushing their way up through the grass, beautiful and sweet-smelling and entirely unchewed by snails, beside a clump of ravishing daffodils with apricot trumpets.

Thursday 15 August

Freezing, torrential rain. House a tip, as it always is on Thursdays after I've been at work for the last three days. James left at six, in the dark, to feed out before a truckful of heifers arrived at the bottom yards. I had to put Blake's lamb down; it hasn't been drinking very well for the last few days, and this morning its back legs were semi-paralysed. Almost certainly a spinal abscess, which should have been prevented by all the colostrum we fed it from birth. Blake is very fatalistic about it and has already chosen a replacement, but Ellie sobbed over the little limp corpse for twenty minutes. I suspect that at least some of her sorrow was engineered to highlight the hardness of her brother's heart.

On the way home from the bus stop (wearing James's old rugby jumper over my pyjamas – lamb euthanasia infringed on personal grooming time) I saw our neighbour Dan's four-wheeler lying upside down at the bottom of the hill. I leapt out of the car into the driving rain, jumped the fence and rushed down the hill. Dan was on his feet, thank goodness – though I nearly knocked him off them when I slipped and had to clutch at him wildly.

'Are you alright?' I cried.

'Yes.'

'What *happened*?'

'Rolled it,' he said curtly, crouching down to peer under the four-wheeler. He stood up again and started trying to heave it back onto its wheels.

I got my hands under the carry tray at the back and helped him.

'Leave it,' he shouted through the downpour. 'You're not dressed for it.'

But I couldn't possibly have got any wetter, so I helped him push the bike up onto its side and then over. It looked fine – nothing bent or broken – but it wouldn't start. I offered to drop him at his cowshed, where he could get some other vehicle, and he said, 'Yeah, okay.'

In the car I asked after his partner, in a last-ditch effort to make conversation, and was told that she's just left him. At which point we arrived at the cowshed, and he got out and walked off without a word.

I got home just as a car full of Jehovah's Witnesses pulled up. We stood at the back door for ten minutes, me dripping and shivering and generally looking like a drowned rat, while Pat Simonson read me selected bits of the *Watchtower* magazine. (This month's caption: *What is God's Name?* Couldn't help wondering why this was an important question.) It was reasonably hard to bear, but Pat is at least 90 and was a friend of James's grandmother so I couldn't tell her to go away.

Saturday 17 August

A beautiful pale-gold morning, with every twig and spider web outlined in dew. James, Ellie and I spent an hour before breakfast doing intensive lamb-related tasks. We moved their pen, put down fresh hay in their little house and barrowed away the old stuff. I spread it around the new trees I've planted down the hill behind the dog kennels, while James and Ellie checked the ewe and two lambs that James is trying to mother up. One of the lambs has caught on; the other is extremely dim and rushes around the ewe in circles, enthusiastically headbutting her armpits in the hope that they'll yield milk. Luckily the ewe has a sweet and patient disposition.

Blake emerged from his bedroom as I came back in to mix up lamb milk, so I told him to put on a jersey and come too. He greeted us at the back door when we returned twenty minutes later; apparently he'd been on the brink of leaving the house when he remembered he really *must* read the latest school newsletter.

Blake is now folding the washing while the rest of us eat French toast.

Sunday 18 August

The nearly dead lamb James brought in yesterday woke not once but three times during the night, and screamed until we got up and fed it. Little bastard.

James came home with three more lambs at lunchtime, bringing the total to eighteen. Two were wild week-old ones whose mother died and who would rather die too than drink milk from a bottle, so I had to tube-feed them while they screamed and thrashed, and one had a joint infection. I should probably have put it down – they don't usually do very well, even after weeks of antibiotics – but it's small and adorable and went to sleep on Ellie's lap.

The children built a fort in Blake's room, using every sheet, blanket and pillow in the house. Then James said something unforgiveable, although I can't quite remember what it was, and I pictured another 40 years trapped in a marriage with someone who neither understands me nor wants to.

At three o'clock I escaped my unsatisfactory family and went for a walk with Amy from next door. I told her all about my horrible day and my mean husband, and she listened and sympathised.

Then she smiled at me very kindly and said, 'So, when's your period due, hon?'

Oh. Tomorrow.

Amy's husband is trying her patience too – and she doesn't have PMS. She's just gone back to work full-time, and she and Sean are taking it in turns to cook dinner. Before they had children, Sean was a great cook, but now he's mysteriously forgotten how. Last night, she said, he hit a new low of tinned tomatoes and tinned corn, mixed together and heated in the microwave.

'What did you say?' I asked.

'I said it was delicious,' she said grimly. 'He's just hoping that if he does a bad enough job I'll take over.'

Monday 19 August

I spayed a cat at work today, the first one in about five years. (A new policy – I am to spend a morning a week doing surgery, thus challenging myself to keep growing and developing while allowing our excellent small-animal vet, who is 67, to have a three-day weekend.) I made a keyhole incision through the flank, as per dim recollection of what I used to do, and then spent fifteen minutes searching with increasing desperation for the uterus. Eventually I decided that she'd probably been spayed already – and, even if she hadn't, I was going to cause internal damage if I didn't stop fishing around blindly in her abdomen – and closed her up again. We turned her onto her back, clipped and scrubbed her stomach, and I made another incision. And there was the uterus, as clear as anything. I had to ring the owner and mentally prepare her for coming to collect a cat with two holes in it. Very awkward phone conversation. Not at all sure about this growth and development thing.

Emerged hot and bothered from surgery to find the others running races. Carrying a 20-kilogram bag of dog food, you had to run around the fibreglass display cow, out through the storeroom, across the car park, around the side of the building, up the road and back in through the front door. Managed to beat Sophie, the new grad, who is sixteen years younger than me – partly because I cut her off and partly because her dog-food-carrying technique needs work but, still, it was encouraging. She doesn't have to make two holes in her cat spays, though.

I was just wondering whether I was a good enough person to go to my Pilates class after work when a calving came in. Excellent excuse. I rang James to tell him I'd be late, and he said he'd started dinner. He'd made bread dough, put some rice on to boil and chopped up some potato and pumpkin to roast. What else did I think we should have? I suggested pasta, for the complete carb suite.

Tuesday 20 August

Heard a most excellent story today from our vet nurse Emma, who is awesome. Her small son electrified his upmarket grandmother recently by saying cheerfully as they all got into the car, 'Buckle up, cunt!'

Nana paled, as well she might, took a deep breath, turned in her seat and asked, 'Where did you hear that word, dear?'

'At school,' he said.

'Do you know what it means?'

'Nope.'

'Well, dear, it means a lady's bottom. It's not a nice word, and it's very silly to use words when you don't know what they mean. I don't want to hear you doing that again, do you understand?'

'Yes, Nana,' he said meekly.

Happiness and reconciliation all round.

The next day Emma got a call from the school principal, flagging his concerns about her son's language. On questioning, the boy explained proudly that he'd told *everybody* at school that a cunt is a lady's bottom, and now that they all knew what it meant, they could all say it.

We mounted a whole-family, military-precision-style operation this evening. Yesterday morning James found a newly dead ewe with two very speedy ten-day-old lambs that he couldn't catch. He couldn't catch them this morning either, but although ten days is old enough to run faster than he can, it's not old enough to be weaned.

We drove out to the paddock on the four-wheeler and found two sad, hungry little lambs snuggled up against their dead mother. I went down the hill to the gate to block off their escape, and James and the kids fanned out across the hillside. We pushed the lambs, as well as another half-dozen ewes, up into a corner, where Blake caught one of them in a fantastic sliding tackle. We left Ellie holding it and re-mustered the ewes and the other lamb into another corner. We hadn't cornered them properly when Blake suddenly launched an attack. He sprinted, he wove, he jinked, he bluffed, he dived – and he caught it! We have no idea where his athletic prowess comes from; I came last in the interschool cross-country every year of primary school and still bear the resulting psychological scars, and at Blake's age James was slow and pudgy.

We bore the lambs home in triumph, and I mixed them each a bottle, with very low expectations that they would drink.

They *attacked* their bottles, and when they'd finished them, they pawed and headbutted us for more. I didn't want to give them too much at once, after three days of starving, but I gave them another little feed at seven, and again at nine. This morning they greeted Ellie and me with wild shrieks of impatience, and they've already learnt how to latch onto the feeder and help themselves. Woohoo!

Thursday 22 August

From where I sit on the couch with my laptop on my knees, I can see a bellbird working his way from flower to flower in the grevillea beside the deck. I hoped that would happen when I planted it – how nice of the bellbirds to comply.

The school cross-country was today. It rained, as it does every year, and we all wondered, as we always do, why cross-country couldn't be held in November instead.

The course crosses the dairy farm next door to the school – down the hill behind the school house, under a fence, onto the race where it exits the cow shed, around the effluent pond, up the next hill and back down a long ridge to the start. Often the next-door farmer, who has a puckish sense of humour, grazes the paddock behind the school house the day before. This year, through some oversight, he hadn't. So no cow pats, although the mud in the race was deep enough to seriously hamper the little ones.

Blake loves cross-country, and ran like a gazelle. Ellie doesn't love it at all, but she ran with grim, long-suffering determination, and actually wouldn't have come last had she not stopped to encourage a flagging new entrant.

I was watching her cross the line hand in hand with little Patrick Fletcher, my heart swelling with love and pride, when my sister-in-law Diane came up beside me.

'There's no way she would have won anyway,' she said consolingly.

The day ended with a House Challenge, and parents were strongly encouraged (i.e. bullied and coerced) to run too. The first house to get every member over the line would be the winner. Under the direction of Shane Ngatai, strategist par excellence, every adult attached to Kereru House carried at least one of the smallest children. I got five-year-old Georgia Martin, who's built like a brick shithouse, and had to stand with my hands on my knees, wheezing, for some time afterwards. But we won. Korimako House, to which my nieces belong, came last. Just saying. (Blake's favourite phrase of the moment. So delightfully passive aggressive.)

Sunday 25 August

Mum and Dad have been here all weekend, which was lovely. We don't see as much of them as I'd like, since they both retired from teaching two years ago and moved to the far north.

My parents are very proud of me. This is almost entirely because I managed to attract and marry James, who is not only a Man of the Land but is, according to my mother, a Delight. I'm fond of him myself, but they take it to ridiculous lengths. If, heaven forbid, I should ever leave him, Mum plans to move in to look after him instead.

We celebrated Blake's birthday in the traditional manner yesterday, with a healthy and nutritious family afternoon tea involving three kinds of chocolate biscuit, three kinds of chip, marshmallows, fizzy drink, sausage rolls and birthday cake. The guests were Mum and Dad, James's mother Val, Thomas, Diane and their two girls, and one of Blake's school friends.

The cake, decorated according to Blake's detailed specifications, was an ocean, heavily infested with sharks and sea snakes. The sharks' fins (royal icing) poked up above the turquoise-coloured waves, and gummy snakes stuck out all around the sides. It looked wonderful, although not particularly edible – there's something sort of off-putting about turquoise butter-cream.

Blake's little friend Keagan smuggled a lamb inside and shut it in Blake's bedroom. Some time later he appeared at my elbow and said, 'Hey! That lamb's pooed everywhere.'

His parents, who I'd thought would drop him off and leave but who instead settled in for the afternoon, thought this was hilarious. They did not offer to help clean up. Instead, I cleaned Blake's carpet while Keagan's father trapped Dad in a corner, accused him of being a bloody left-wing Labour voter like all teachers, and told him that the proposed new Emissions Trading Scheme, which will allow big businesses from overseas to buy perfectly good farmland and plant it in pine trees to offset their emissions, thus destroying rural communities, was entirely the fault of greenie arseholes like Dad.

James and Thomas talked about farming, as they always do. Thomas is two years older and four inches shorter than James, with more hair but a chronically worried expression. He doesn't talk to me; when we come face to face, he looks panicky, nods, mutters 'g'day' and rapidly retreats. I like to think this is due to extreme shyness rather than extreme dislike, although this has never been properly confirmed. I used to ask James from time to time if his brother liked me, and he always said, 'What? Why wouldn't he?' which was only marginally reassuring.

Mum and Val went into a huddle on the sofa with a glass of wine each. Val hardly ever drinks and she went all pink and giggly. Very cute. Mum told me later that Val's seeing someone, but it's very early days and she doesn't want the children (us) to know about it. How lovely – it's time Val met somebody nice. James's father died very suddenly five years ago, of a heart attack.

That left Diane sitting dumbly at the table with Keagan's mother, Cheryl. They have absolutely nothing in common. I tried for a while to think of topics of conversation, but it was uphill work. Eventually, in desperation, I suggested we go outside and look around the garden.

Neither of them looked at all enthusiastic about this idea, but they came. We traversed the lawn in silence, broken occasionally by me saying inane things like, 'Ooh, look, a bellbird!' and, 'Isn't it a gorgeous time of year?'

The kids were all down in the lamb paddock below the orchard. As we reached the fence a dozen lambs bounced up to us, turned tail and raced away in a crazy game of tag. Ellie's pet lamb was asleep on her lap and Diane's eldest, Rachel, was sitting high up in the big copper beech. The boys and my second niece, Holly, were shrieking with laughter as they turned forward rolls down the hill. We stood beneath a plum tree arrayed in gorgeous bridal white, surrounded by drifts of daffodils. The sky was clear and blue, the air warm and fragrant. And Cheryl said, 'I hate living in the country.'

'That's a shame,' I murmured weakly.

'You write books, don't you?'

'Yes.'

'I started writing a book a few years ago.'

'Did you? Cool! What's it about?'

'Oh, it's just based on my own life. No-one'll ever publish it; they only publish mass-market crap these days.'

I wasn't sure how to reply to that, so I said nothing.

'I'd send it to you, but I don't want to give away my ideas.'

I hastily told her that she was very wise.

Diane then remarked that she saw a picture of me in the local paper and barely recognised me. It was a *lovely* photo, she said. I looked so *young*. I've changed *so much* since it was taken.

I took them back inside and retreated to the couch with Mum and Val. There are limits to a hostess's obligations.

Wednesday 28 August

It's half past eight, and I've gone to bed with the laptop to write some deathless prose (or, more likely, a couple of hundred mediocre words that will be passable after half-a-dozen revisions; let's not be unrealistic). But I can't concentrate at all and am struggling to resist the urge to check Facebook, which will inform me only that everyone I know is doing something more exciting than I am and that more orangutans are dead after the felling of another piece of rainforest.

No. Must write. Perhaps I'll start by writing down what I did today, as a warm-up exercise.

5.15 a.m. Woken by very loud purring on the pillow beside me. Pushed cat off bed. Cat returned fourteen seconds later. Pushed cat off again. Cat returned.

5.16 a.m. James got up, removed cat, closed bedroom door and returned to bed.

5.23 a.m. Lay awake thinking about how James is a better person than me and I really should have done that myself. Moved on to thinking about the wonderful opportunity to get some writing done that I was wasting. Bed suddenly became a thousand times softer and more comfortable than it had ever been before.

5.31 a.m. Guilt at lying in bed increasing. Began speculating on how long it had been since I woke James up to have sex with him. Couldn't remember. Poor sign; would not like marriage to fail through apathy and lack of effort. On the other hand, too comfortable to move.

5.38 a.m. Woke James up. James surprised but enthusiastic. Most gratifying.

5.58 a.m. Got up and moved to couch to write.

6.42 a.m. Writing going swimmingly.

6.45 a.m. to 8 a.m. James got up and started mixing lamb milk. Shut down computer, put on load of washing, fed sick lamb in laundry. Lamb not looking great despite 36 hours in intensive care. Tubed it and gave it various drugs. Went outside to help James. Bottle-fed nine smallest lambs, brought in bigger lambs' feeders to clean. Cleaned and refilled them, took them out, got dressed, attempted to beat hair into submission while Blake hovered in the hall asking for popcorn in his school lunch. Made popcorn. Told Blake to have breakfast and empty his lunchbox from yesterday. Cleaned lamb bottles. Made marinade and massaged it into tonight's roast. Hung out washing. Discovered Blake had rested a plastic bag on the hot element while filling it with popcorn. Shouted a little. Attempted to remove melted plastic from stovetop. Brushed Ellie's hair and did it in an asymmetrical French plait like Prim's in *The Hunger Games*. Handed James coffee out the window. Hung out washing and put on another load. Asked children to help tidy up – Ellie wiped down a bench; Blake folded a tea towel. Discovered he had neither made his lunch nor had breakfast, and that we had to leave the house in three minutes.

8.02 a.m. Dropped children at the bus stop and continued on to work.

8.30 a.m. to 3 p.m. First job this morning: sedate menacing dog and spay it. Dog a mastiff–Shar Pei cross and approximately the size of a bear. Luckily the dog control officer is fantastically brave and held the sharp end while I jabbed it. While we waited for the dog to go to sleep, dog control officer told horror stories of dogs that have attacked him. Spayed dog. Resisted temptation to overdose it with anaesthetic and make the world a better place. Spoke at the counter to a woman who dragged four wild baby rabbits out of their burrow yesterday to be pets for her preschoolers. One had died after being carried around all afternoon. Suggested its death was due to intense and prolonged stress, and that constant handling wasn't good for baby rabbits. She replied that if the children couldn't play with the rabbits there was no point in having them, and asked if there were any diseases rabbits could give to children. Managed not to say 'I hope so' out loud. Castrated another, much nicer, dog. Went to see a calf with an abscess on its jaw. Lanced abscess – very satisfying. Returned to clinic and spayed a cat, accompanied by Counting Crows, thanks to Emma the world's best vet nurse. Victory: only had to make one hole in the cat. Went to see a down cow on my way home. Cow at the back of the farm; had to ring Amy and ask her to collect my children as well as hers from the school bus.

3.15 p.m. Passed section of broken fence on my way up the road and car lying on its side in our bull paddock. Jaide was in attendance; the driver had just left her house, very drunk. She had already called the police. Driver of the car was sitting in the paddock humming a little tune. Rang James, who was down at the pump. James slightly curt due to inability to fix the pump and having already been rung and told about the fence by two other people.

3.50 p.m. Continued up the road to collect children from Amy's place.

4.10 p.m. Reached home at the same time as Jaide, who was calling in to give me the drunk driver's name and phone number. Drunk driver is her sister's boyfriend, and calling the police has led to major family discord. Jaide tearful. Gave her a cup of tea.

4.45 p.m. Jaide left. Fed lambs. Sick lamb greatly improved. Brought in washing.

5.20 p.m. Realised I'd forgotten to put mutton in oven. Got out sausages instead and put them in hot water to defrost.

5.30 p.m. Admired Blake's ball-kicking skills. Helped him climb onto the roof to retrieve his ball. Picked a bunch of daffodils while waiting to help him down again. Forced both children to shower and wash their hair.

5.47 p.m. Sausages into oven. Threw potatoes, pumpkin and silverbeet into a pot to boil.

(Unexpectedly delicious if mashed together with sufficient cheese, even though it looks like somebody already ate it.) Remembered baking for tomorrow, to be dropped at the accountants as a thankyou from the swimming club for doing their accounts for free. Decided to give accountants half the chocolate cake I made yesterday. Found seven-eighths of it already eaten. Started – muttering – to make another one.

6.05 p.m. James appeared at the kitchen window and handed in five kilograms of venison back steak, covered in grass and hair, from a deer he shot on the way home. Very pleased with himself. He also brought home the deer's head and propped it against the back tyre of the ute, where it will no doubt stay until I move it.

6.08 p.m. Phone rang – had forgotten I was on call – to summon me to a calving on the other side of town. Delighted to leave James to deal with steak, dinner and cake. Thoroughly enjoyed drive to calving, calving itself and drive home. Very restful.

7.40 p.m. Got home. Had dinner. Read Blake a chapter of *The Horse and his Boy* and discussed Lucius White from school, who told Blake that Jackson and Keagan don't want to be his friends anymore when actually they do.

8.10 p.m. Snuggled Ellie up. Discussed the crimes of Mrs Denny the cooking teacher, who explains things so slowly that everybody's bran muffins

were still raw in the middle by the time they had to catch the bus.
8.20 p.m. Showered.
8.30 p.m. Bed with laptop.

Hmm. No wonder I'm tired. I'm going to sleep.

Thursday 29 August

I dropped the cake off at the accountants on my way to the dentist this morning. It was whisked away by a woman I didn't recognise, which was a little deflating. Now neither the swimming club nor the accountants will ever know that I did my duty.

I was much more deflated five minutes later, when Amy rang my cell phone to say our rams were on her lawn. Totally my fault – I called in at the woolshed for petrol this morning and forgot to shut the road gate. I had to ring James and get him to go and sort it out. He was right at the back of the farm. He explained, not nastily but at somewhat wearying length, how important it is to leave gates the way you find them.

Got home to find an email from my publisher asking if I'd like to record the audio version of my latest two books. In Melbourne! If so, could I record myself reading the first few pages of the book and send the file through for the audiobook people to listen to? Immediately recorded the sample and sent it off. How cool!

Saturday 31 August

Interesting things we have discovered while giving lambs their last feed, after dark:

- Clover leaves fold up for the night like little books.
- Spiders' eyes glow green in the light of a head torch. If you look for the tiny emerald stars you find all sorts, from great velvety brown water spiders to tiny translucent ones, mooching around in the grass engaged in various arachnoid pursuits.
- The other night James and I happened upon a nocturnal worm soiree. I don't know what they were up to – a worm orgy? – but as we came back across the lawn after feeding the lambs, it was absolutely *seething* with worms. As we approached they whisked themselves below ground much, much faster than I thought worms could move, so that the grass in front of us was a shifting, glinting mass of disappearing worm tails.

Spring

Spring to me means lambs and calves and new baby leaves uncurling and the world growing steadily greener and fresher and lovelier until I think, 'Ah, yes, spring is officially here now. Very pretty.' And then every plant puts on six inches of lime-green or gold or copper-coloured new growth, and it isn't just pretty, it's spectacular.

Spring is never quite getting on top of the lawn, and wondering every night I'm on call if this is going to be the night the after-hours phone rings at 11.30 p.m. with a calving an hour's drive away, and then rings again at 5 a.m. for a prolapse.

It's ducklings on the main pond and tuis in the kowhai tree and quail chicks the size and shape of bumble bees. And plum blossom and daffodils and wave after wave of spring flowers, each brighter and frothier and gaudier than the last.

I really, really love spring.

Monday 2 September

I don't expect farmers to hover around me obsequiously when I turn up, or help me to clean my gear, but it's nice when they bother to say hello.

I went out to a farm to calve a cow this afternoon. Two people in the vicinity: one hosing the yard and the other feeding calves. 'Hello!' I called. No reply. I got out my drug box, my calving bucket and my lube pump, and lugged them up the steps to the shed. The farmer ceased hosing and came to watch me thread my way around and through the bars – it's an old-fashioned rotary shed and you've actually got to climb through the pipework to reach the race on the far side. He didn't relieve me of any of the things I was carrying.

I asked what the problem was. He said he thought it was twisted. I said it was nice to see the sun for a change. He said, 'Mm.' I remarked – but he was gone.

It *was* a twisted uterus, a condition resulting from a big, sprightly calf turning cartwheels and taking the whole uterus with it. Uterine torsions come in various degrees – with a complete twist the vagina is completely closed off, like the neck of a bread bag you've twisted shut, and you have to cast the cow with ropes and roll her across the ground, hoping that the uterus will stay put as the cow rotates and it will all come back into alignment – but if you can reach the calf you can sometimes flip it back the way it came and unwind the uterus from the inside.

I could just get my hand through the vaginal canal and reach the calf's nose. I held his head – he didn't like it much, and kept tossing it pettishly – and pushed him away from me as I swept him down and around clockwise. It's bloody hard to flip over 40 kilograms of wriggling calf at arm's length, working through a tight, crooked tunnel.

He struggled and writhed and generally made a nuisance of himself for a few minutes – just enough to really tickle up my tennis elbow – and then, with a wriggle and a kick, he slowly rolled himself over. The tight band of tissue around my arm miraculously released, the cervix was wide open, and there was a nose and two front feet in front of me. There's nothing quite like the heady sense of accomplishment that gives you.

I must admit, in fairness, that at this point the farmer and his neighbour, who had just dropped in, wandered over and pulled on a leg rope each. The calf came out without a hitch. They let the cow out of the front of the race and wandered off again, leaving me to collect all my gear, thread it back through the pipes, wash it, pack it up and carry it back out to the ute. I wrote the docket and climbed back through the obstacle course to give it to them, whereupon the farmer said, 'Eh?', scribbled his initials across a corner and turned his back on me.

I drove away feeling slightly aggrieved and returned to the clinic, where I discovered that our senior vet Melissa's terrier, who is very cute but has no class whatsoever, had been whiling away a happy half-hour while the vet room was empty by chewing the lids off four specimen pots containing faecal samples that were waiting on my desk to be tested, and licking out the contents. Wasn't sure whether to laugh or throw up.

Wednesday 4 September

Current lamb count is 26 – twelve in the big mob, ten slightly younger ones and four babies on the lawn. The oldest twelve are totally uninterested in us now, except as the bearers of a bucket of milk twice a day. This includes, unfortunately, Ellie's and Blake's lambs for Pet Day. James decreed on Sunday that they be separated from the mob and penned up on the lawn to be hand-fed, but they hated it so much we couldn't bear it and put them back in with their friends. This afternoon I ordered the children out of the house to spend quality time with them – at *least* fifteen minutes. No, you may not finish your computer game level first. Well, if the grass is wet, wear your waterproof trousers. Yes, you *do* have to go to Pet Day. Because you'll regret it on the day when your friends are all having fun outside and you have to stay in class and do maths, that's why. And because perseverance is the most valuable trait a person can have, and you're going to learn some, so help me God ...

Amy says she's taken to locking her children outside rather than embarking on these long and painful arguments – they beat at the door and sob for a few minutes, and then wander off and play. I think I'll try it.

The deer head is still beside the ute, at the front door. It's been there for a week. I could move it, but I feel that would be a moral victory to James. Will continue reminding him to do something about it. That worked with the old Holden Commodore with lichen on the windscreen that lived on the lawn of our first house. It only took him three years.

Friday 6 September

After school this afternoon, prompted partly by the realisation that we hadn't seen Nana for a week and partly by the hope that there would be something delicious in her tins, the kids and I went to see Val. She lives two kilometres up the road, next door to Thomas and Diane, in a beautifully renovated cottage. When her husband died, she decided that she was tired of rattling around in the big homestead (I suspect she was also tired of Diane's artless comments about the inadequacy of her own home), and swapped houses with Thomas and Diane. She had most of the cottage's internal walls taken out and all the windows enlarged and double-glazed. Then she polished up the old rimu floorboards, previously hidden beneath mustard-coloured carpet, and painted the walls a soft eggshell blue. It's gorgeous.

There was another car there when we arrived, a shiny black SUV. Inside we found Trevor Cartwright, a big, happy man with a booming laugh who's been selling real estate for 30 years.

Val wasn't nearly as pleased to see us as usual – she was pink and flustered, and told me twice that Trevor was an old family friend who'd just popped in *completely* out of the blue.

While we were eating ginger gems Val told me that Thalia is coming home with her fiancé next month. Thalia is Thomas and James's baby sister. She's 29 and has been in England working as a project manager for the past five years. I've never quite grasped the intricacies of her job, except that it seems to involve drinking champagne at Ascot and entertaining various CEOs on yachts while sailing around the Greek Islands. She's lovely (and she has many fabulous shoes, which fit me); it will be wonderful to have her home again.

Sunday 8 September

Just finished reading a book in which a couple who have been married for 30 years attribute the success of their marriage to their passionate and highly experimental love life. Really? After 30 years? Can't help reflecting that the most exciting recent development in our marital bed has been James's discovery that he sleeps much better if he wears socks at night to keep his feet warm.

Wednesday 11 September

Ridiculous day at work. Just ridiculous. Ridiculousness made considerably worse by my own disorganisation, which is extra galling.

I left home just after seven to be at a distant farm by eight, feeling highly efficient. Arrived on farm at seven fifty-five. No cows. The dull-eyed youth hosing down the yard said, in response to my question, that the boss was at the other farm this morning; the vet was coming. The other farm was 45 minutes away, a mere 20 minutes from home.

Frantically radioed the clinic – no-one else was free. Drove across the district, arriving three-quarters of an hour late. The farmer was sweet and understanding, but I felt like a twerp.

Returned – late – to the clinic to start morning surgery. Castrated two goats and a basset hound. Drove back to the end of the district I'd already visited by mistake to calve a beef cow. The cow was on a hill at the back of the farm, tied to the tractor with a strop around her neck. She was understandably annoyed about that, and because the strop was three metres long, she had a lot of room to move. The calf was coming tail first, and I got the back legs up while trotting backwards and forwards in a half-circle as she plunged at the end of the strop – which I thought was quite a good effort. The farmer didn't look particularly impressed, but he's the cranky type who fears that saying something complimentary might increase the bill.

I returned to the clinic to pick up Sophie, and we set out to vasectomise ten bulls. There were twenty-three in the yard when we got there. 'Just do as many as you can,' the farmer said. We got pretty efficient – five bulls into the race, vaccinate, blood test and sedate all five, let them through one by one into the head bail, vasectomise one testicle and castrate the other, move on to the next. We did fifteen in three hours, by which time we were well and truly over it. One of the first bulls we did worried us by dripping blood in a thin but relentless trickle from his castration wound – we watched him for an hour in the hope it would stop and then got him back in and sewed his scrotum tightly shut. Then we watched for another hour as the scrotum grew bigger and tighter and fuller of blood, hoping that the pressure would stop the bleeding rather than grow so great that the stitches burst and the bull collapsed in a lake of blood. That's the sort of thing that really keeps you alert and interested in your work. (It stopped. Thank God.)

We finished the Vasectomy Marathon in time for me to meet the school bus – but there were several urgent calls backed up. I rang James, who said he could meet the bus, and went to see a sick cow.

The sick cow had a displaced stomach and needed surgery. It was three forty-five and my surgery kit was soaking in a bucket at the clinic. Returned to get it and found Sophie and Bill embarking on de-constipating a badly constipated dog (constipated dogs always arrive after four; it's an unalterable constant in an ever-changing world). I scrubbed my kit at lightning speed, rushed back to the side of the cow, sedated her, roped her down, rolled her onto her back, made a hole in her abdomen, deflated the offending bit of stomach, stitched it to the body wall so it couldn't go astray again, sewed her up, woke her up again and left.

Got home at quarter to seven. The smell of rotting venison greeted me as I climbed out of my ute. I replied to my husband's cheerful greeting by snarling, 'Either that bloody deer's head goes or I do.'

James did not respond, as he might have, by pointing out that I was four hours late home and had entirely stuffed up his afternoon. Instead he said, 'I promise I'll take it away in the morning,' and handed me a glass of wine. Decided my mother is right; he is a Delight.

Thursday 12 September

I DIDN'T HAVE TO GO TO WORK TODAY! And it was a beautiful, warm spring day, the sort where everything is lush and green and you can practically see the grass growing.

James left early, and I fed the lambs by myself. This consists, on the new ad lib system, of mixing up two ten-litre buckets of milk, wandering outside and tipping one into either feeder. This time last year we would have been filling individual bottles and feeding a dozen lambs at a time, in shifts. I *love* the new system.

I paused on the way back in to note that my pink tulips with electric blue middles are flowering their little hearts out, and that there were fourteen tuis feeding in the kowhai tree. Mrs George Huthnance, an especially luscious rhododendron, is just coming into creamy peach-tipped bloom.

Inside I found Blake up and making his lunch. Should he wake Ellie? I agreed, and almost immediately heard loud wails from Ellie's room. It turns out she doesn't like to be woken by being shot in the head with a Nerf gun. Who would have thought? Blake's defence: he wasn't there at all, he missed her completely and he only shot her very gently anyway.

Having decided that today was a wonderful opportunity to write, I instead spent two hours reupholstering a chair with red-and-gold-striped brocade. It would look amazing if Bean the cat hadn't immediately decided I'd done it just for her to use as a scratching post. The chair is now covered with a blanket, which we'll be able to remove when Bean dies. This may be quite soon.

Friday 13 September

This morning at the bus stop Jaide told me all about her sister (not the one whose boyfriend drove through our fence; the other one) and her problems. The sister has four children with four different fathers. She left the father of the smallest one (who is nine months old) in July, after hooking up with his friend at a party. The friend has several children himself but isn't allowed to see them unsupervised due to a history of family violence. Two weeks after the sister moved in with him, he beat her up. Now she and the children are staying with Jaide, and the sister is very unhappy, because although her partner hit her, he's actually the love of her life and he didn't really mean it. Came home feeling very, very privileged and middle class and clueless.

Saturday 14 September

I've been looking through an old cookbook Mum found at a book sale. It is endearingly titled *Mary Bought a Little Lamb and This Is How She Cooked It*. It's fascinating. It contains not one but two recipes for liver paste (a tasty sandwich filling, apparently – who knew?), suggests creamed lamb with sautéed cucumbers for a dinner party and makes multiple references to adding a teaspoon of MSG for flavour. I made the mutton hash for dinner, because it contained neither sautéed cucumber nor MSG and because mutton hash features in *Dear Enemy*, which is one of my favourite books of all time. It was delicious. Perhaps I should be brave and try the liver paste. (But I won't.)

Sunday 15 September

Our wonderful neighbours arrived this afternoon with two calves on a trailer, one each for Ellie and Blake. They used Speckle Park bulls over their herd this year, and the calves are extremely cute: white with black noses, thick black eyeliner around their eyes and black teddy-bear ears. They'd never been let out before, and they ran excited laps around the little paddock below the yards with their tails straight up in the air.

The neighbours are going to leave a bucket of milk for them at the end of the driveway every morning, asking only that we leave yesterday's empty bucket as a swap. They are far, far too generous, but they were so happy, and so obviously delighted at the kids' delight, that we couldn't refuse.

The lambs are now just despicable little woolly white things in Ellie and Blake's eyes. They spent all afternoon with the calves and would have slept with them if we'd let them. I anticipate this fervour to last about three days, after which they will return to their normal state of grumbling and muttering when asked to feed their pets.

Monday 16 September

I've been invited to speak at a literary festival in Wellington in November. Just like a real writer! The festival organisers will pay for my flights and hotel room, and I'll have all day Sunday free to hang out with my friend Kelly, who lives in Wellington. How wonderful.

Or so I thought until I received a summary of the events in which I would be participating.

The first is a high tea, during which another author and I will discuss our latest novels. The other author is really nice and really funny and has a regular radio slot, so the audience is bound to be entertained even if I can't manage to say anything useful. But the second event! It's entitled 'Women's Bodies: Conflict Zone', and the clarifying email from the woman chairing it explains that the aim will be to explore what it means to be in a woman's body these days, with reference to the 'invasions of privacy, abuse, claustrophobic attention, readings and misreadings, clamps on how we feel we're allowed to exist, think and behave', and so on, that we are subjected to as women. Each author on the panel is to interpret the broad idea in a way that works for her and her writing.

Bloody hell.

That is *so* not my cup of tea.

I know that women – some women – are subjected to all sorts of horrible things, but I haven't been. I *don't* feel that my body is a conflict zone, or that being in a woman's body subjects me to any particular invasions or misconceptions. (That's not to say that I think sexism and the gender pay gap and magazines telling girls they should be slim and beautiful aren't real issues – they are real, and they suck.) But all this Conflict Zone stuff just strikes me as melodramatic and whiney.

I wrote back to the organisers suggesting that perhaps I wasn't a good fit for this event, since their whole approach kind of put my back up. To which they replied very graciously, saying that was fine and I was welcome to approach the subject from a positive point of view.

What on earth am I going to say?

Thursday 19 September

It was raining steadily at breakfast time. The cold that's been circling all week launched a full-on offensive overnight and I woke up feeling like I'd been beaten all over with a stick. After getting the kids onto the bus I took two Panadols and shuffled back to bed. Then I lay there for half an hour wondering why my heart was racing and my eyes wouldn't stay shut. Got up again and tottered out to the kitchen, where I discovered that I had taken Panadol Extra, which is laced with caffeine, instead of normal Panadol.

I retired sourly to the couch with my laptop, where I found an email from my publishers informing me that the audiobook people have given my voice 'the thumbs down' and will be using an actress instead. Ouch. I don't know what's wrong with my voice, and suspect that enquiring would only depress me further.

Got up off the couch and started scrubbing the laundry floor, on the grounds that I might as well wallow in misery while I was at it. A year ago, we replaced the ancient and horrible lino in the laundry with new stuff, selecting a hard-wearing, black-and-white check. It did not occur to me at the time to make sure that the new lino was non-absorbent. In fact, had I thought about it, I would have assumed that all lino was non-absorbent by definition, seeing as the whole *point* of lino is that you can just wipe it clean. But this stuff is porous, and cleaning it requires scrubbing on your knees with Jif and a stiff brush.

I was halfway across the floor when someone knocked on the back door just behind me and scared me out of my few remaining wits. I struggled to my feet and opened the door to find our friendly neighbourhood Jehovah's Witness, Mrs Simonson. She was beautifully turned out, with her silver hair immaculately set and a pale-green silk scarf around her neck. I was in flannelette pyjamas with uncombed hair and a red nose, clutching a scrubbing brush. (I suppose it could have been worse; I could have been clutching a bottle of gin.)

She greeted me with her usual sweet smile, opened this month's *Watchtower* and read me an article assuring me that Hell is Real. I had no trouble at all believing it. Then we chatted about farming for a little while, and she told me how pleased she and her husband were to sell the rest of their silage last week. Apparently, it's dreadful silage – it was rained on twice before being baled – so they were thrilled to sell it for a top price to some lifestyle-blockers who know no better. I said I didn't think that was a very Christian thing to do (which was tactless, but I was feeling pretty lousy), and she looked at me with a sort of amused pity. 'That's *business*, dear,' she said. Oh. Right. That's okay, then.

Friday 20 September

My cold had loosened its death grip on my sinuses by this morning, and the sun was shining. The tui count in the big kowhai outside the kitchen window was 43.

James and I docked two paddocks of ewes and lambs before lunch, and it went surprisingly well. I find performing farm jobs under James's direction somewhat stressful – he's so bad at giving instructions. I never know what the plan is, and if I ask he either says he told me already but I didn't listen (there may be a grain of truth in this), or he looks at me with withering scorn and says it should be obvious. Which might also be true, but is hardly helpful.

Last year I came across an article in *Countrywide* magazine that I found very reassuring. It was written by a charming and immensely capable woman who said that her husband, although otherwise quite satisfactory, has on occasion been such a dick in the yards that she's downed tools and walked home, taking the dogs with her. Thank heaven it's not just me.

My idea of a happy marriage has changed quite a lot in thirteen and a half years. I started off thinking that ideally your husband should be your soul mate, your lover, your best friend and your sounding board, that he should understand everything about you and love your every flaw.

Rubbish. Complete crap. One person will *never* fulfil your every need and want and desire for the rest of your life. The thing to do, I have come to realise, is just accept that my husband feels that $100 is too much to spend on a pair of shoes, thinks *Dumb and Dumber* is the funniest movie ever filmed and can't see why his standard response to any apology ('That's okay, but [insert detailed reiteration of whatever it was I did wrong, just to make really sure I get it]') is annoying *at all*, and move on. Better to remember that he's a wonderful father, he makes me a coffee every morning and he buys me a Pixie Caramel every time he does the grocery shopping.

But I digress. Today was reasonably harmonious, although James did feel the need to give me a few tips on how to improve my lamb-vaccination technique. I have, after all, only been a large-animal vet for nineteen years. He picked up the lambs and vaccinated them for scabby mouth, and I jabbed them with 5 in 1, castrated and cut off tails.

I don't mind cutting the tails so much – of course it hurts them, but the pain doesn't seem to last very long and the docking iron cauterises as it cuts – but I *hate* putting rubber rings on scrotums. You go out to muster them away and see the poor little things lying down and rolling in agony. I'd roll in agony too, if someone put a rubber band around my finger and waited for it to fall off. But this year a lovely drug rep has given me two big bottles of pain relief gel specially formulated to use at docking, in the hope I'll be so impressed with it that I'll recommend it to every farmer I meet. I will, I think. Today's lambs didn't look *entirely* happy, but it must be an improvement.

In the afternoon I stayed home and wrote, and James went out to move heifers. He met Dan – our dairy farming neighbour whose girlfriend recently left him – on the road, and invited him to dinner. Unfortunately, dinner was lentil bolognaise, which is not really the sort of food one wants to offer a guest (at least not a guest one wishes to return).

To give him credit, Dan tackled the lentil bolognaise gamely. He even had seconds. Then, when the conversation touched for some reason on Jehovah's Witnesses, he told us that they haven't been to his place for two years. On their last visit they came to his front door while he was having lunch, and on the way to open it, he noticed he'd left his shotgun leaning against the wall. He picked it up in one hand and gave the door, which sticks in damp weather, a mighty tug with the other. The Witnesses took one look at him, turned tail and fled. He said he tried to call after them and explain, but they were having none of it. He actually smiled while recounting this story. The smile transformed him from sulky and nondescript to boy-next-door charming.

Goodness, he's nice. I wonder if I could organise for him to meet Sophie at work, who is feeling, at the ripe old age of twenty-six, as if she's the only single person in the world and she's going to die alone, eaten by her many cats. She only has two cats – but, as she says grimly, they're a start.

Sunday 22 September

On call this weekend. It's been fairly quiet – which is a blessing because on Friday night I gouged a hole in my hand with my eye hook.

Eye hooks are smallish (about the size of a bent finger) and bluntish, and are designed to fit securely into the eye socket of a dead calf so you can apply traction to the head. I don't use mine very often, but Friday night's calving was the sort where every instrument gets dragged out of my calving bucket in turn.

The cow had a twisted uterus; a complete twist, so I had to rope her down and roll her. The twist unrolled alright, but the calf was still upside down and I could only just reach it with my arm at full stretch.

I put ropes around the front legs and then managed, barely, to get a rope around the lower jaw. (Calving textbooks tell you that the lower jaw isn't a good anchor for a rope, and you should place your head rope around the back of the calf's head behind the ears. Well, yes. You should. And you would, if you could reach that far.) The rope slipped off when I pulled it, as jaw ropes mostly do, but at least it brought the head ten centimetres closer, so I could just reach an eye socket.

I placed the eye hook and connected it to my calving pulley. Mistake number one. And because the damn head was still upside down, wanting nothing more than to bury itself inextricably beneath the brim of the cow's pelvis, I kept my arm in the cow to try to turn it as the farmer applied traction. Mistake number two. As the farmer hauled the rope tight the hook pulled free of the calf's eye socket and embedded itself in the palm of my hand.

I couldn't see the wound properly, but there was a lot of blood welling up from under the torn edges of my glove. The farmer showed no interest in my injury – I wasn't expecting him to kiss it better, but he could have said, 'Are you alright?' and given me the chance to be impressively brave. But he just stood there waiting for me to do something useful, so I put my hand back in – trying not to dwell on the fact that the calf had been dead for a couple of days and I was bathing my open wound in a bacterial soup – and found that the head was now close enough to put a proper head rope on.

Once the calf was out, I left my gear in a pile on the yard and inspected the wound. It was quite impressive: deep and jagged and four centimetres long. I poured neat iodine all over it, on the grounds that gangrene would be no fun at all. The iodine wasn't much fun either, just quietly.

I'd rather hoped that the farmer might have started washing my gear, since I only had one working hand. But no; he was just standing there looking at his phone. In desperation I asked him to hose off my casting rope, a soft, thick, eight-metre-long cotton rope and he said, 'Oh. Sure,' and dribbled some water on it. Jeez.

However, I got everything packed up alright and called in at the clinic on my way home to put on a proper bandage. I found a little pot of local anaesthetic gel, used for painting calves' heads after dehorning, and dripped some into the wound. It worked a treat. I never felt another twinge all night, and I calved two more cows on Saturday and one this morning with no trouble at all.

Monday 23 September

I found Ellie crying in bed tonight. She said it was nothing and that I couldn't help anyway, but eventually she told me that the other girls at school aren't talking to her, and when they play four-square they gang up to get her out as quickly as possible.

'Which girls?' I asked.

'It's mostly Hannah, but then Rachel and Temeira join in.'

I never did like Hannah. Uppity, sour little brat. And as for Rachel, what else could be expected from a child of Diane's?

'How long has this been going on?' I asked.

'All this term. But please don't do anything, Mum, *please*.'

I promised not to (although I may break this promise and have a quiet word with her teacher), and we got out my phone and listened to 'Mean' by Taylor Swift. Ellie seemed slightly consoled by the fact that even Taylor Swift had to deal with this shit. Then I kissed her goodnight and went away, seething.

How can I fix it? Should I even try to? If I leap in, will it make her think that this is a really big deal and she should be really worried? It was so much simpler when she was a baby and it was clearly my job to protect her from everything bad.

Tuesday 24 September

While making myself a cup of coffee this morning I lost focus while pouring in the hot water, overfilled the cup and burnt my hand. The same hand I sliced open with an eye hook. 'How can you *possibly* get distracted pouring hot water into a coffee cup? It's a two-second job,' said James. I told him that it was because my mind is on a Higher Plane. He looked doubtful and said, 'Yes, maybe, or perhaps you just have the attention span of a goldfish.'

I called Ellie's teacher this afternoon between small-animal consults. She told me she's never seen even a *hint* of discord or trouble among the girls in her class – they're a delightful group – but she *completely* understands how difficult it is for parents. It's *totally* natural for parents to be overprotective, and children – perhaps girls especially – are just a *teensy* bit prone to exaggeration. Mostly these things turn out to be mere tiny blips. She'll keep a close eye on things, although of course she keeps a microscopically close eye on things anyway. I'm trying hard not to feel patronised, and failing.

Wednesday 25 September

Disaster! Cathy Mitchell is coming to stay! We were in the same year at vet school; not really friends, but in the same social group. We had bugger-all in common – I wanted nothing more in the world than to be a large-animal vet, while she thought that Art, Culture and all good things were confined exclusively to cities – and we never kept in touch after we graduated.

She contacted me via Facebook a few weeks ago, far more warmly than our acquaintance warranted, and like a fool I replied in a similar vein. She suggested it would be lovely to catch up sometime, and I replied, *Absolutely!* As you do. To which she responded: *Yay! How about next week?*

James says that if I don't like her, why did I invite her to come and stay? I find this unhelpful.

Thursday 26 September

I dropped the kids off at the bus this morning and carried on into the middle of the farm to dock. I got there just as James got the mob into the back of the yards. It was a beautiful morning – soft, cool breeze; tiny puffy clouds in a cornflower blue sky; aspen trees along the track covered with tiny, translucent, pink-gold new leaves. When we went to muster in the second mob we saw a duck nesting in a hole in a tree two metres above the ground, with just her beak poking out. I wonder how she plans to get the ducklings down when they're born.

There was a moment of tension at the gate into the yards, when the mob broke and Taz the huntaway, who is nine years old and really should know better, chased the escapees enthusiastically in the wrong direction. We lost two lambs through the fence into another mob, which means James will have to mix them all up so they can find their mothers again, but luckily there was no possible way that it could have been my fault. I toyed briefly with the idea of explaining to James why it would be better if his dogs were properly controlled, just to see how he liked it for a change, and decided it wouldn't be worth it. As Ursula le Guin (I think; it may have been someone else equally wise) once said, the key to a successful marriage is leaving about half-a-dozen things a day unsaid.

Friday 27 September

Blake's class had an end-of-term party today. He tells me they ate chips, marshmallows, gummy bears and miniature chocolate fish. Which is very nice, but I can't help thinking it's a puzzling contrast to the stern notes the school sends home from time to time, reminding parents that junk food in lunchboxes is *not* appropriate.

Another thing I find contradictory is the karakia that precedes every school morning tea and lunchtime. Bible in Schools isn't taught anymore, on the grounds that it's inappropriate to promote Christianity at the expense of other religions. Well, fair enough. In my Bible in Schools classes we just made papier mâché camels and cooked our very own Middle Eastern flatbread, but other teachers may well have been less fun and more fundamentalist than mine.

But if saying grace in English is offensive, why is it fine to say it in Maori?

I just went down the hall and found one naked child stuffing the other out of a bedroom window. Both were laughing uproariously, so I decided it was best not to intervene.

Sunday 29 September

I am trying to write and help Blake make a chocolate cake at the same time. Very fragmenting to the attention. Here is a small example:

> B: Can I make mince pie?
> Me: Sorry, love, we have no mince. (We're subsisting on lentil bolognaise while waiting for Murray the steer to grow big enough to eat.)
> B: Ooh, Mum, how about orange chocolate muffins?
> Me: No oranges.
> B: Chocolate muffins.

Me: Yes!

B: Where's the recipe?

Me: Inside the front cover of my recipe book.

B: This one?

Me: That's not my recipe book.

B: This one?

Me: Yes.

B: Where's the recipe?

Me: Inside the front cover.

B: Where?

Me: Inside the *front cover*.

B: Here?

Me: That's not the front cover.

B: This one?

Me: That's a recipe for chicken teriyaki, Blake.

B: Oh. Here it is, Mum! I found it!

Me (wearily): Well done, love.

B: Three teaspoons of instant coffee ... Is this a teaspoon, Mum?

Me (with slight edge to my voice): What do you think?

B: Um, yes. So how much do I put in? Isn't it great that I'm helping you, Mum, so you can write?

Tuesday 1 October

Blake and I finished *The Lord of the Rings* this evening. Not just the story, but all the appendices. He wouldn't let me skip a single list of Númenórean kings. Anyone who wants to know anything about the history of Middle Earth up to the end of the Second Age should see me.

I've been contemplating murder today. Not maliciously, but because I spent an hour with a man who is such a blight on the planet that I really think it would be best to put him down.

This stain on the undies of society is in his fifties, with horrible teeth, and has a rough, steep little farm miles out of town. He comes into the clinic occasionally to lean on the counter and unsettle poor Jess the receptionist, who is young and pretty.

I went out to his farm today to see a lame bull. It had a dislocated hip that had never been put back in and had formed a false joint. Absolutely nothing to be done about it, six months down the track.

The grass on his farm is so short it's like a fine green scum. There's a formerly lovely wetland beside the track, now a chewed-out mud puddle. He's been digging ugly channels through it with a bulldozer. (I surmise, from the way he spoke of 'those fucking cunts at the regional council', that they do not approve of this course of action.)

He explained to me that it doesn't matter when he puts the rams out; the lambs come at exactly the same time of year anyway. I suggested that perhaps he had some stray rams, but he rejected this obviously moronic notion; it's because of something in his soil. Good to know.

Then he told me at length about his plans to properly break the place in. He has several hundred acres of native bush, and just as soon as he can afford to, he's going to spray it out and turn it to good grazing land. The horrible bastard. I told James about it when I got home and he said I shouldn't worry; it's actually really expensive to spray out bush and he'll never be able to afford to do it. But what if he realises that and burns it? No, I really think killing him is the best option.

Thursday 3 October

Today was gorgeous; cool and crisp in the morning, and warm and balmy after lunch. The garden is full of lovely flowers – from the kitchen windows I can see bluebells and Dutch irises and sparaxis and clematis and rhododendrons and freesias – and all the things that lose their leaves in winter are putting out new ones, so clean and bright and perfect that it makes you want to compose an Ode to Spring, or at least an Ode to Baby Viburnum Leaves. Gangs of tuis, having torn the last flowers off the big kowhai tree, are mooching around the garden picking on the bellbirds to pass the time while they wait for the rewarewa trees down in the bush to come into flower.

Both children had friends over; the girls put in a couple of hours of extensive calf training while the boys put in a couple of hours making an enormous blanket fort in Blake's room, with the windows, doors and curtains firmly closed. A perfectly logical way of spending the nicest day for weeks. Anyway, all was happiness and laughter, especially when I made them cinnamon doughnuts for lunch.

In the afternoon I dug the boys out of their blanket cave and made them come down the farm with me to spray a patch of tradescantia that's spreading up from the creek bank through the bush with terrifying speed and determination. On the way home we saw the duck that nested halfway up a tree. I assume it was her, anyway; she was in the pond beside said tree. She had a line of nine ducklings behind her, so they must have managed the descent without mishap.

Friday 4 October

Cathy Mitchell arrived this afternoon. She has swingy, shoulder-length, caramel-coloured hair and sculpted upper arms, and she was perfectly, beautifully made up. I felt dowdy and weather-beaten by comparison, and I'm sure I looked it.

She talked until bedtime without stopping, about her Sydney apartment and her job (the boss is jealous of her and undermines her constantly) and her personal trainer and her wonderful new man. She's on a gluten- and dairy-free diet so couldn't eat the chicken pie I'd made for dinner. She showed no interest at all in the children, and looked faintly pained whenever one of them spoke. I don't expect visitors to fawn over the kids, but they do live here, after all. When we said goodnight, both James and I begged her to seize the chance to have a really good sleep-in tomorrow.

Saturday 5 October

Cathy rose at nine and had a long shower, which gave us a nice peaceful stretch of time to get the calves and lambs fed and the housework done. As soon as she emerged, James, who had been drifting around cleaning the dog kennels and halving grapefruit for the tuis, suddenly realised he urgently needed to spray gorse at the back of the farm. (Oddly enough, he was seized by the exact same realisation when my aunt and uncle last stayed.) Ellie and Blake went up to Val's on their bikes, and I spent an hour sitting at the kitchen table hearing about Cathy's ex's new girlfriend, who is a fiend in human form.

An hour of that was all I could take, so I dragged her out to check the stoat traps around the edge of the bush. The tally was one stoat and three hedgehogs – I was delighted; I hardly ever get a stoat – and Cathy remarked that she'd always believed a vet's vocation was to *save* animals. I was so irritated that I subjected her to a lecture on the terrible depredations of stoats on native birds and of hedgehogs on native insects, which bored her stiff.

After lunch the kids escaped to the calf paddock and James escaped to tidy up the woolshed. Cathy and I went out into the garden, where I weeded while she talked. It was a lovely afternoon – even she noticed, and leant back on her wrists with a sigh, saying, 'Your life is so peaceful and stress-free.'

I said, 'Well, yes, sometimes,' and she told me that I had no idea how tough things are for other people. Which is perfectly true, except that she didn't mean people in Sierra Leone or Aleppo, she meant herself. It really annoyed me, so I asked whether she knew I'd spent all of the year before last being treated for breast cancer.

'Oh, well, I –' she started, but I didn't even let her finish the sentence. I told her how, after weeks of biopsies and scans and ultrasounds, we were told that the lump in my breast was a malignant carcinoma that had spread to the local lymph nodes, and how James, who I'd only ever seen cry when his father died, burst into tears in the hospital car park. I had five months of chemotherapy that, as well as killing cancer cells, did horrible things to my stomach lining, made all my hair fall out, including my eyebrows and eyelashes, and induced early menopause. Then I had a mastectomy and about 30 lymph nodes removed, and a twenty-hour breast reconstruction surgery. The reconstruction failed because my veins were in such lousy shape from the chemo, and they had to remove the new breast again two days later. I spent a week in hospital and another three weeks shuffling around at home with a walker and three big bottles collecting fluid leaking from my drain sites. Then I had a five-week course of daily radiotherapy. There were ongoing complications at the wound site and I spent another week in hospital on IV antibiotics. It took me months of exercises to get back the range of movement in my right shoulder, and it still aches at night. Without clothes on, I look like I've been attacked by a shark.

'God, that's awful,' Cathy whispered.

I said it's not awful; it's the *complete opposite*. I'm cured. It's all over, and I get to forget all about it and carry on with my life.

'That's, um, great,' said poor Cathy. She was thoroughly cowed, and only began to revive under the influence of wine. I may have overdone the rant.

Sunday 6 October

Cathy left this morning to have lunch with a friend on her way to the airport. I think she was as pleased to leave us as we were to see her go. I wonder why she wanted to catch up in the first place? Had she forgotten we have nothing in common, or did she just have a couple of days to kill? We docked the pet lambs – we should have done it weeks ago – and I planted the potatoes. There was no room for them in the veggie garden, which I planted solid with chicory and Shirley poppies last autumn. A few leeks are struggling gamely through the poppies towards the light, but I haven't seen my garlic for months.

I know perfectly well that planting potatoes in the flower garden leads to digging them up and cursing for the rest of your gardening life (my aunt, whose family had a potato fight in her garden twenty years ago, is very vocal on this subject), but I chose not to think about that, and tucked them at the back of a border between a climbing rose and a patch of Shasta daisies. Oh well.

Tuesday 8 October

My first work call this morning was to a down cow with, the farmer said, a twisted gut. He's been farming for 30 years, and he knew as soon as he saw it that this cow's problem was more than simple milk fever. So he left the bottle of calcium he'd intended to give it on top of a fence post and called the vet.

I examined the cow – very cold, heartbeat so faint I couldn't hear it (although she must have had one; she was sitting up), kink in neck, dry nose, not dehydrated, no mastitis – and said I thought it was milk fever.

'That's not just milk fever,' he insisted. 'I've been farming for thirty years.'

I gave her the bottle of calcium he'd left on the post, and she burped and shivered and started looking like a live cow instead of a frozen one. I gave her another bottle, and her neck straightened out and I could hear her heart again.

The poor man was crushed. I told him everyone makes that mistake, and I only learnt from making it myself to always, *always* give down cows calcium, even if you don't think that's the problem.

He wasn't consoled, so I told him about the incident last week where I sent a bloated puppy to a specialist for further work-up. The specialist diagnosed overeating. The farmer laughed for longer than I felt was strictly necessary.

Wednesday 9 October

My peerless and wonderful mother-in-law has given me a whole box of bulbocodium bulbs – little gold petticoat daffodils, ten centimetres tall. I spent an hour this evening planting them all through the orchard, where next year they will dust the soft spring grass like little flakes of gold. At least that's what they'll do in my imagination, which is where my garden schemes are usually at their best.

Friday 11 October

I've been feeling frustrated about my lack of writing time, so I got up at five thirty this morning to get some done.

James got up at five forty-five and sat down across the kitchen table with his new book on World War II. He told me that when Germany invaded France, they came through the Ardennes forest, which was completely unwatched and unprotected because the Allies thought nobody in their right minds would bring battalions of tanks along its narrow, winding roads.

'Gosh,' I said.

Five minutes' quiet.

'Hey, this is interesting.'

'Mm?'

'Did you know that although seventeen thousand American troops lost limbs in combat, a *hundred* thousand American civilians lost limbs over the same period in industrial accidents back home?'

'Wow.'

'And –'

'Love, I'd really like to get some writing done.'

'Sorry,' he said stiffly.

Seven minutes of silence.

'Far out,' said James.

Long pause. 'What?' I asked.

'Doesn't matter.' He was practically quivering with suppressed information.

'No, tell me.'

'Did you realise France had had *forty-two* weak governments between 1920 and 1940? No wonder their morale was in the toilet.'

'That's amazing. I had no idea.'

'Me neither. Hey, do you want another coffee?'

And so it continued until it was time to start mixing lamb milk. It's lucky I like him.

Thomas came down this afternoon for some drugs to treat a calf with a swollen knee. He wouldn't come in, and he wouldn't have an apricot danish (I made some as an experiment, and they're *awesome*). I got him some anti-inflammatories and antibiotics out of the back of my work ute, and he grunted at me and left. I wish Thomas liked me. He's so nice to other people.

Saturday 12 October

The carminia, a very classy rata vine, is flowering in the bush below the house. It's bright crimson and covers about a quarter of an acre. It's gorgeous.

Ellie biked up to see her grandmother this afternoon and returned with a hideous vase shaped like a mermaid's tail, a set of framed prints of smudgy watercolour pansies and a cellophane-wrapped basket of virulent purple gift soaps. I do wish Val wouldn't use our house as a repository for useless and horrible crap unearthed while clearing out cupboards – but then she did give me that box of bulbocodiums.

Clare rang this evening to ask how I am.

'Um, fine,' I said, slightly perplexed. 'How are you?'

'Oh, fine. Same old. I just heard from Suzanne that you're in a bit of a dark place at the moment, so I thought I'd better ring up and check.'

'*Suzanne?* I haven't talked to her for months!'

'She was talking to Cathy. Apparently you're really struggling since your cancer treatment.'

I told Clare all about Cathy's visit, with particular emphasis on her extreme self-absorption and the dairy- and gluten-free diet which didn't stop her eating a huge hunk of chocolate brownie after her carefully prepared dairy- and gluten-free dinner. We had a lovely time picking the poor woman to shreds. We also planned a girls' trip to Waiheke Island, where Clare's brother has a house, for a weekend at the end of November. James has given his blessing (that sounds like I'm a doormat); we won't be weaning or shearing, so he won't need me. I can't wait.

Sunday 13 October

Blake arrived home from his friend Keagan's house this evening with a baby pigeon in a box. They 'rescued' it – that apparently being what you call climbing to the top of a hay barn and removing a baby bird from its nest. It's the ugliest thing I've ever seen: covered in grey fuzz with an enormous, bulbous purple beak that looks both faintly indecent and three sizes too big for it. On asking YouTube how to feed baby pigeons, we learnt that they don't open their mouths for you to put things in; their mothers stick their heads down the babies' throats and regurgitate partly digested food directly into their stomachs. So glad I only had to lactate. I made a delectable mixture of pureed porridge, peas and corn kernels. Then we watched a video – posted by a pigeon fancier from Wisconsin called Al – that showed us how to simulate a mother pigeon by filling a jar with pigeon porridge, stretching a rubber glove tightly over the top, making a little hole in the glove, poking the pigeon's beak through and turning the jar upside down. It actually worked! He gulped quite a lot, and went to sleep on Ellie's lap.

Monday 14 October

I took Pidge to work, where he was met with universal cries of disgust. Disappointing, from a whole building full of supposed animal lovers. I spent the morning palpating non-cycling cows. (To palpate a non-cycling cow: Insert arm up to shoulder into cow's rectum. Locate ovaries through rectal wall. Plump, knobbly ovaries suggest cow has ovulated or will shortly; miserable jelly-bean-sized ovaries mean she hasn't and won't. Treat jelly-bean-ovaried cows with progesterone.) Then I rushed back into the clinic to feed Pidge, and rushed back out to spend two and a half hours standing on a cold and draughty platform in an ancient rotary cowshed, probing the vaginas of the blue-painted cows with a little rubber cup on the end of a stick as they went past. This is done to find and treat any uterine infections before mating, and is even less fun than palpating non-cycling cows. I can't imagine the cows enjoy it either. About one cow in ten was painted blue and the platform moved as fast as a snail can crawl. If they'd drafted the blue cows out at morning milking it would have been a 30-minute job to check them, but we charge per cow rather than per minute, and it didn't bother the farmer to have me standing there for hours. Thank goodness for the Kindle app on my phone – I read half of *The Book of Dust* between cows, and although it wasn't the most comfortable way to read, it saved me from going mad with frustration.

When I got home, I went out to bring in the washing and found Ellie reading in the paddock just over the fence, propped up against one calf and with the other at her feet. School was okay, she said. The girls were calling her Smelly Ellie, but she pretended not to notice and read her book. I went back in and left a message on the school voicemail asking the principal to ring me.

Tuesday 15 October

At work this afternoon we had a call from the other practice in town. Someone had brought in an old and very sick tabby cat with one white forepaw they'd found wandering in the car park at a local bush reserve. The fur over the veins in its forelegs were clipped, so they thought it must have recently been seen by a vet and wondered if we might remember it.

We did. It sounded just like Taffy McGee, a lovely cat we've been treating for diabetes. So I rang Mrs McGee, a tiny, sweet, frail lady in her eighties, to ask if Taffy was missing.

'No, dear,' she said. 'Taffy's been put to sleep.'

'Oh, I'm so sorry, I didn't realise,' I said, thinking it must have been on a day I wasn't at work.

'That's fine, dear. It nearly broke my heart, but it was just too much for me to manage her injections, with my husband so unwell, so I got my son to bring her in and have her put to sleep two weeks ago.'

I got off the phone and checked our records. No visit since 20 September, when we checked Taffy's blood glucose level and renewed the prescription for insulin. I asked the others – no-one had put Taffy down and forgotten to update the computer.

I called back the opposition and said the cat I had in mind had apparently been euthanased. But would they mind just checking the blood glucose of the cat they had in the clinic?

They wouldn't mind. Their cat had a blood glucose level of 45, which is *way* above normal. She was nearly comatose, and they put her down.

I'm so angry with that useless rotten son I could kick him. He took an old, sick cat, who slept on her owners' bed and had a little bit of salmon every night as an entree, and abandoned her in the bush to die slowly of diabetes and/or starvation. Was he just saving himself a dollar, or did he actually think that he was being kind?

Wednesday 16 October

With extreme cunning, I organised for Sophie the new grad to go out and palpate our neighbour Dan's non-cycling cows today.

It's not, I admit, the most classically romantic setting for them to meet, but having them both for dinner would be excruciatingly obvious and embarrassing. On her return, Sophie reported he was a nice guy and they had a good laugh, which sounds promising.

The school principal rang me back. She's never seen any sign of strife between the older girls – they're a bouncy, happy, high-spirited, inclusive group of girls (it sounds like they were all created by Enid Blyton) – but, yes, she'll keep an eye on things.

James and Blake are practising goal kicks on the lawn in the soft spring twilight. I just went past on my way to the washing line and pointed out, with commendable mildness, that they've snapped off three fat lily shoots in the neighbouring garden bed. This was greeted with cries of: 'Oh no, the Muminator is on the warpath!' 'She looks mad!' *'Run!'*

I stalked back inside, followed by James, who made me a gin and tonic to appease me. I'm ashamed to admit that it worked like a charm.

Thursday 17 October

We are bidden to a family dinner at Val's this Saturday – Thalia and her fiancé are flying in at some ungodly hour tomorrow night. It will be wonderful to see them both. I'm bringing cheesecake and potato salad, and Diane's doing nibbles.

I tried to make falafels for dinner. James gets all misty-eyed when he talks about eating falafels in Turkey, when he backpacked through the Middle East with the girlfriend before me, back in the golden days of his youth. Epic fail. The falafels (and the girlfriend, I'm pleased to say), not the trip. The mixture looked good and tasted good, but when I shaped it into nice little balls and dropped them into boiling oil they dissolved. Instead of a heap of luscious, golden-brown falafels, I ended up with a pot of oily chickpea sludge.

Ellie and Pidge are inseparable. She carries him around on her shoulder and he sleeps on her pillow. In the mornings he wakes her by climbing her face and gently pecking her eyelids until she opens them. Which is quite cute, apart from the tiny, insignificant detail that pigeons are a bit like small winged cows and poo more or less continuously. Ellie addresses the problem by covering her bed with towels – this results in having to wash several towels as well as her duvet cover every day. I am going to have to put my foot down and insist Pidge sleep in his box, even if it breaks his heart and Ellie's.

Saturday 19 October

We just got home from Val's place and tucked the kids into bed. James doesn't want to talk about the evening. 'Their business, not ours,' he said, oozing moral superiority from every pore, and turned on the rugby highlights. James can be very annoying at times.

It's a blow, because I'm *dying* to talk it over, and writing it down comes a poor second.

However. We went up to Val's just after five. Thalia and Adam were there – Thomas picked them up from the airport at four o'clock this morning – and we were still in the initial It's-so-awesome-to-see-you-and-the-kids-are-all-enormous-and-can-Adam-honestly-play-music-through-his-*sunglasses* stage of conversation when Trevor Cartwright arrived. That was surprising, and it became rapidly more surprising when Val – *Val*, who never rocks the boat or does anything that might possibly upset anyone – took him firmly by the hand, led him to the edge of the deck (the rest of us were on the lawn below, so it was like a balcony appearance by the Queen) and said, 'Everybody! Quiet, please. I think you should all know that Trevor and I are lovers.'

There was a long, excruciating silence, and then James muttered, 'Good stuff, Mum,' and everyone talked feverishly about something else.

It's lovely that Val has found someone nice. I couldn't be happier for her. But what would have been wrong with the traditional approach of saying nothing and leaving your friends and relations to join the dots in their own time?

In other news, I was heading next door to borrow some baking powder from Amy this morning when I met Dan on the road. After discussing grass growth (slow) and mating (good despite shortage of grass; twelve cows on heat this morning), he asked if I could see to it that in future he doesn't get that new girl when he needs a vet. She was nice enough but a bit indecisive. No offence, he knows new vets have to learn, he'd just rather they didn't learn at his place.

Bugger.

Sunday 20 October

The biggest and fattest of the pet lambs was dead this morning. Twisted gut, I expect, poor thing. But why must lambs die after they've drunk $100 worth of milk powder? Could they not do the decent thing and die at birth, if die they must? Just saying. It's especially inconsiderate to die at the bottom of the hill, not the top – I dragged the corpse up and heaved it onto the back of the ute, and then had to sit down for a while and gasp for breath.

Thalia came down after breakfast, bearing an absolutely ravishing mint-green chiffon shirt dress that she says was a mistake, with her colouring. It isn't with mine – at least, I hope it isn't, and it's so beautiful I don't care if it is. She told James that she thinks he looks even better without hair and Ellie that Pidge is obviously a bird of great personality and charm, agreed with Blake that his hair looks just like Beauden Barrett's and said my last book was her absolute favourite, equal with all the others. Such a nice contrast to Diane's take-'em-down-a-peg-or-two approach.

We went out to admire Ellie's calves, and as we came back up through the orchard Thalia stopped under an apple tree, grabbed my arm and said, 'I'll do *anything* if you'll let me get married in your garden in February.'

I told her that wouldn't be necessary, and of course she can get married in the garden if she wants to. It would be an honour.

It was only later, after what Jane Austen refers to as a period of quiet reflection, that several things occurred to me:

1. My garden's nice now, but by February it looks pretty tired and dusty. I am not one of those

geniuses whose gardening year is a constantly unfolding progression of loveliness, with every plant's post-flowering scruffy stage hidden by its neighbour's moment of glory.
2. Thalia is a perfectionist. Her goal is flawlessness; mine is to have things pretty good some of the time.
3. January and February are crazy months. There's a huge amount of sheep work to be done – shearing and dipping and dagging and drenching and sending lambs to the works – and it's my busiest time at work, too. We usually make hay, and there's usually some major disaster with the water reticulation system. We also like to try to get away on holiday for a few days, so our children's memories of summer don't exclusively involve sheep yards.

Oh, shit.

Monday 21 October

It's 11.30 p.m. and I'm in Dunedin, tucked up in my Airbnb bed, looking out through a floor-to-ceiling window at the city lights below. I'm very relieved to be here – an hour ago it looked like touch and go.

Tomorrow is the annual Veterinary Parasite Advisory Day, when the country's best and brightest parasitological brains convene to talk about drench resistance. I love worms and drench resistance, and I've always wanted to go to Dunedin, but what a mission!

I had to leave work at four at the latest to get to the airport, and my last consult was a dog with a chronic ear infection and atopic dermatitis. Skin cases are complicated and time-consuming at the best of times, and the lady was a talker. I dashed out of the building at 4.07 p.m., and heard myself being paged for a final boarding call as I ran through the automatic doors at the airport. Whew.

We changed planes in Wellington. I read the boarding time on my ticket wrong (apparently I have yet to master the 24-hour clock) and thought I had an hour and a half. So instead of grabbing some dinner I wandered into a bookshop, where I found that the New Zealand fiction section contained every book published this year except mine. I was dragged from my depressed contemplations by the boarding call, and rushed through security, where they confiscated the pocketknife my grandmother gave me when I was ten. The knife blade was short enough to pass, but the saw was three millimetres too long. Well, gee, fair enough. You never know when some crazed passenger might try to stab the pilot to death with a Swiss army knife saw blade. I tried to explain it would take quite a lot of sawing to reach a vital spot, even assuming the pilot sat quietly while you tried and nobody else noticed what you were doing, but they obviously feel that you can't be too careful. They wouldn't hold the knife for me to pick up on the way home, and there's no post office at the airport, so it's gone for good.

We got to Dunedin at nine, and I caught a shuttle into town. It's a shame it was dark and raining, because I'm sure we toured the entire city and I'd have got a wonderful feel for the place.

Eventually the shuttle stopped halfway up a very steep, very dark street, and I got out. I found the right number with the light on my cell phone and headed down a long driveway, stepping in several puddles. The room was in a concrete apartment block behind a big red-brick house, across a building site and up three flights of steps. I explored the building site for some time before finding the right steps, and then up I went, found the lockbox for room 3B and opened it with the code I'd been given. There was no key in the lockbox.

I found the room and tried the door – locked. It was after ten by then, and raining quite hard. I called my hostess, waking her up, and explained that I couldn't get in. She talked for a long time about the uselessness of the cleaners and how desperately unfair it all was, which annoyed me slightly, since I was the one standing in the rain. But eventually she groaned and said she'd come down with the master key.

She arrived ten minutes later – ten minutes feels like a long time when it's raining and six degrees and you didn't pack a jacket – and opened the door. The room hadn't been cleaned after the last occupants left, so the bed was unmade and the sink full of dishes. We stripped the bed and made it up again, and she said unenthusiastically that she could refund me the night. I'd probably have told her not to bother if she'd been pleasant, but she wasn't, so I said, Thank you, that would be great.

So now I'm in bed, warm and comfortable but too hungry to sleep. Oh well, apparently intermittent fasting is terribly good for you.

Tuesday 22 October

Great day. Parasites are fascinating. I've learnt that fourteen days is the optimal time between samplings for faecal egg count reduction tests, and that *Haemonchus* stage-four larvae are inherently quite resistant to levamisole, and various other terribly useful facts that I scrawled on the back of the program and will hopefully be able to decipher later. I've also caught up with several nice people I hadn't seen for years. I'm supposed to be having dinner with some of them – but it's dark and it's raining, the restaurant's a ten-minute walk away, and I could just put on my pyjamas and eat the baguette and butter I bought for breakfast on the way back to my room. That would be very feeble and unsociable, though …

Bugger it, the rain's getting heavier. I'm texting my apologies and staying here.

Wednesday 23 October

It wasn't raining this morning – well, not much – and I had time to walk around the Botanic Gardens before the conference started. The rock garden is *gorgeous*; all full of gentians and pulsatillas and tiny irises that I can't grow at home because it isn't cold enough.

Hmm. I couldn't be bothered going out for dinner last night, with several witty and charming people whose company I enjoy, but I had no problem getting up at 6 a.m. to walk around a garden in the drizzle. Worrying. I quite like the idea of becoming charmingly eccentric as I get older, but what if I'm just turning into an unsociable weirdo? James will be no help in preventing it from happening; he's not very sociable either.

Another full day of parasites. Mostly very interesting – worms are so cool – except the last presentation, where someone explained a recent study which found that some dead newborn lambs whose mothers were treated with drench capsules have high levels of abamectin in their brains, and some don't. No information was forthcoming as to what causes this variation – or, indeed, what, if any, concentration of abamectin in the brain is toxic. It was a very labour-intensive study, and apparently they got half-a-million dollars of government funding to do it. The whole exercise seems to have been a colossal waste of time and money. I suppose at least they did no harm – years ago a zoologist friend told me about a study where some sadistic PhD student attached little heart rate monitors to Adélie penguins and made them run on treadmills until they collapsed. (That was in America, where getting ethics approval for cruel and pointless experiments seems to be quite easy.)

I remembered to get dinner at the airport tonight, and had a spectacular view of the Southern Alps as we flew up the east coast of the South Island. I sat beside a nice man who's investigating a new and delicious lure for stoats (Hooray! *Useful* science!) and got home just after nine. Ellie never stirred when I crept in to kiss her goodnight, but Blake smiled, shot upright, threw his arms around me and cried, 'Mum! You're home! Yay!' Most heart-warming.

Thursday 24 October

Diane called in to borrow the water blaster. She said she's had a terrible time with scours in the orphan calves, but she got some great advice from the Farming Mums Facebook page and now it's all sorted out. Well, why would you ask your sister-in-law the practising farm vet when you could ask Facebook?

We had parent–teacher interviews down at school this evening. Blake, we were told, is a model student. He's very bright, he's pleasant and attentive, he helps the other students and his hard work and perseverance are classroom watchwords. I checked, and no, there was no mix-up, she *was* talking about our child. Crikey. Of course we like Blake quite a lot, but at home he is not renowned for his hard work and perseverance – he's famous for oozing quietly away whenever you'd like a hand with something.

We floated out of Blake's classroom and into Ellie's. There we learnt that she's a great kid; that although her maths could be improved there are no real concerns with her learning; and that they've had words with a couple of the senior girls who were throwing their weight around, and the feeling in the staffroom is that things are much better.

That's our feeling too. Hooray!

Friday 25 October

I strayed into Mitre 10 this morning after doing the grocery shopping and accidentally bought a cornflower-blue salvia and a beautiful white peony. They jumped out and accosted me as I went past on my way to the vegetable seedlings. Especially the peony; it was so glossy and sturdy and fresh, with half-a-dozen fat buds. But driving home I remembered that a peony needs a good square metre of rich, sunny, fertile soil all to itself, that all my sunny spots are already full of other things, and that I have killed more than one peony in the past by pretending it would be perfectly happy jammed between two large shrubs in dappled shade. Not wanting this one's sap on my hands, so to speak, I carried on to Val's place to give it to her.

She looked at the peony, looked at me, said, 'Oh, *sweetie*! How *lovely*!' and burst into tears. Then she straightaway apologised for being so silly.

I sat down at the kitchen table and asked what was wrong.

Nothing at all, she said. Just foolishness. Just that she's been unkind and insensitive and upset everyone and spoilt Thalia's homecoming.

'Rubbish!' I cried, but she just smiled sadly.

I said that she couldn't be unkind if she tried, and there's no way she's spoilt Thalia's homecoming, and if anyone is upset that she's happy they're obviously so selfish that being upset is just what they needed. And then I added, because she didn't look convinced, that James, for one, was *delighted* that she was seeing Trevor.

'What did he say?' she asked.

'"Good on them",' I said promptly, and she started to look quite cheerful.

It *wasn't* a lie. He might not have put it in those exact words – or in any words at all, if we're going to be all pedantic about it – but of *course* James wants his mother to be happy. And since he'll never, ever discuss the subject with her, I am safe to interpret his feelings on the matter as I see fit.

Saturday 26 October

At lunchtime James played me a wonderful old interview with Barbara Cartland, which he randomly encountered on a podcast about Viking history. Dame Barbara produced a book a day, reclining on a couch and speaking into a dictaphone. She despised women as being vastly inferior to men, and said that if your husband leaves you it's your own fault for not being sufficiently alluring. (I wonder if she actually believed that, or just said it for the shock value?) She served tea and cake to her little dogs before allowing her guests to eat and had her butler 'exercise' the Rolls by driving it around in circles in front of the house. I can't decide whether I think she was ghastly or fabulous.

Either way, she certainly has me beat for output. I got up at five this morning and spent two hours writing 100 words and deleting 150.

Sunday 27 October

Oh, dear Lord. The All Blacks lost the World Cup semi-final to England. Decisively. England totally deserved to win; they were unstoppable. But losing to England is so much worse than losing to anyone else.

Monday 28 October

Melissa, who is English, came in early to work this morning to stick a picture of Owen Farrell (captain of the England rugby team) to everyone's computer screen. She found the perfect picture for the job – he's got an insufferably smug expression on his face. So has Melissa.

Wednesday 30 October

Today was one of those days where everything goes wrong – not disastrously wrong, just wrong enough to spoil your temper. I'm sure it's easier to remain serene in times of real crisis than it is to laugh off a stream of minor irritations. (I may not think so if I was having a real crisis, of course.)

We cut the lambs down to one feed a day yesterday. They protested by biting the ends off half the rubber teats on the feeder, so when I went down this morning and poured the milk in, it cascaded out again in every direction, including straight down my gumboot. Right then, that's it; they're now weaned.

I backed my work ute into a post and dented a panel. Again.

I forgot my lunch. And it was such a nice lunch – rice pudding made with coconut cream and stewed plums.

There was a vet nursing student seeing practice at work – very intense, very keen – who followed me around while I was doing surgery, getting in the way and asking inane questions. ('What's that?' 'The bladder.' 'What would happen if you cut it by mistake?' 'The urine would all leak out into the abdomen.' 'What would happen to the cat then?' 'It would die if you didn't sew up the hole again.' 'You'd better be really careful, then, hadn't you?' 'You don't say.')

I went out to vaccinate calves for a sweet but desperately disorganised farmer. The facilities were poor and the calves had never seen them before. They had to be pushed into the race one by one, and then pushed out of the gate at the front. While I vaccinated them, he drenched them, treated them for fly and castrated the bull calves. His drench gun was broken. The mobs got mixed up. He asked me to look at his old dog while I was there. It was a fifteen-minute job, and it took an hour and a half.

I rang Goldpine to find out whether they'd got in the fencing staples they didn't have last week – they hadn't, there are none in the country, and they're not making any more. Ever. We are, however, welcome to trade in our staple gun for a new, up-to-date model, costing a mere $1400.

I rushed home from work, leapt from my work ute to the car, flew down to school, picked up the children and drove for three-quarters of an hour to get Ellie's eyes tested (she remarked a couple of weeks ago that she couldn't read small writing). Our appointment isn't today, it's tomorrow. They couldn't fit us in, and the receptionist explained to me at length that it couldn't possibly be her who made the mistake. I expect she's right, but I feel that more tact and less insistence on her part would have been nice.

We went to the Warehouse to find white shoes for the children's end-of-year dance concert (we've already paid $50 apiece for their costumes; the white shoes are extra). We found some for Ellie – fairly nasty and more expensive than I'd have liked – but none for Blake. As we went in, I saw a frumpy, greying woman on the security camera, and realised with a jolt that it was me.

All very discouraging, but on the other hand when we got home James was frying potato cakes. And when I was tidying the living room before bed, I found a used envelope on which Ellie had written: *Mum is amazing at most things.* What a tribute!

Saturday 2 November

James's uncle and aunt, truly delightful people, came to see us today. Aunty Cass brought fairy cakes with rainbow sprinkles, homemade sausage rolls, a quiche and biscuits shaped like bats for Halloween. I used, once, to feel a bit aggrieved as I put the nice things I'd made for lunch into the fridge and laid theirs out instead. Did Cass think that if she didn't bring food there wouldn't be any? But now I'm older and slightly more sensible, and I'm just grateful. It's a much better approach.

When they left, James filled their car with boxes of sirloin steak (we tired of lentils a fortnight ago and decided that Murray the steer was big enough to eat). It's wonderful that James is such a warm and generous person, but at this rate we'll be back to lentils by Christmas.

Sunday 3 November

James and I went out for dinner last night with friends we hardly ever see. They have two share-milking jobs and three teenage girls, each of whom have about half-a-million after-school activities. Also, Duncan runs a farm discussion group, Sarah works four days a week off farm, and she's doing a social work degree by correspondence. I have no idea how they do it all without having twin nervous breakdowns.

I think last night is the first time we've got together without our children since any of the children were born. Their two eldest came to our wedding. We were all a bit giddy with the excitement of it – we had entrees and mains and desserts and coffee, whether we wanted them or not, to make it last as long as possible. We left reluctantly when the staff started putting chairs on tables. At one point we were joined by a man who farms near Duncan and Sarah. He explained gleefully that he'd just got the restaurant manager, whom he'd met before, to guess what his name was, *and the manager had got it wrong*! We were all to address him loudly as Nigel to maintain the deception. This wasn't a problem, since none of us could remember what his name actually was.

I woke up this morning with my head pounding as if I'd been drinking hard all night. It seemed unfair, when I only had two glasses of wine. I think it must have been a food hangover, brought on by crab patties, hoisin duck and cardamom cheesecake.

The headache was still there when we went out to drench a mob of lambs after lunch. We could only find one working drench gun, so to start with I drenched and James made suggestions about how my technique could be improved. Eventually I snarled, 'Why don't *you* drench and I'll tell you what *you're* doing wrong?' Whereupon he smiled sweetly, took the drench gun and did a much better job than I had done. Has he no tact?

We had left the children at home, and got back to find Blake uninterested in dinner and with a sore tummy. Just sore, he said; he didn't feel sick. Which wasn't very reassuring, as Blake never does feel sick until two seconds before he throws up, and he's a champion projectile vomiter. I tucked him up with a sick bowl and a hot-water bottle then retreated to the kitchen, where I discovered that of the twenty bagels I made this morning, only eight remained. I hadn't had any, James had eaten one and Ellie two. Nine bagels is probably quite a good explanation for a sore tummy.

Monday 4 November

South Africa won the rugby World Cup. No pictures of smug English rugby players in the vet room this morning; Melissa was very subdued. I considered finding a picture of that South

African player with the flowing blond Fabio-esque hair and slipping it into her diary – but no. I'm not man enough to start a prank war with Melissa. She has a better imagination than me, and much more stamina.

This morning I asked Blake if my work shorts looked alright or if they were too tight. He looked at me thoughtfully for a while and said, 'You look fine, Mum, just a tiny little bit fat.' He then continued, as I hastily took the shorts off again, 'You know what, Mum? Why don't you grow your hair like Aunty Diane? You would look pretty. Not so scruffy.' Self-esteem currently at rock bottom.

Wednesday 6 November, 5.30 a.m.

I didn't sleep very well. I have a doctor's appointment this afternoon to check out a tiny, insignificant lump in my armpit that I'm almost positive is just a little bit of scar tissue from my cancer surgery. It's probably been there ever since, and I just didn't notice. But the oncologist explained to me at the time that if my cancer *did* come back, it would be incurable. They've already hit it with chemo and surgery and radiotherapy; there isn't any other treatment.

I'd forgotten how scary it is, wondering. I've been perfectly certain I'm fine for the last eighteen months, and now I'm only *almost* certain. Cancers recur. It happens. And as soon as you say plaintively to yourself, 'Not me. Surely not. I've done my time,' you remember that things just happen, and it doesn't make any difference at all whether you deserve them. Why *not* me?

I wish I hadn't written it down. It's made it real.

9 p.m.

The doctor is 99 percent positive it's a little bit of scar tissue. But she's referring me up to the breast care unit at the hospital so they can make absolutely sure. In the meantime, I'm not to worry. She was very kind about my hypochondriac tendencies, and although I feel a bit silly, I also feel very relieved.

I scared James as well as myself, which was a shame. He sent me a kissing emoji at lunchtime (his usual text message style tends more towards *Remember drench* or *Dog food x 2 please*), requested a phone call as soon as I left my appointment, and answered on the first ring. He came home at four o'clock, which is unheard of, and played cricket with the kids on the lawn until dinnertime rather than using valuable daylight hours to spray Californian thistles or batten a fence. The game was a stop-start affair, owing to Pidge launching himself off Ellie's shoulder from time to time and landing on the crease. If we raise that pigeon to adulthood without standing on it or allowing Bean to eat it, it will be a miracle.

I was the crowd, going wild when anyone got runs or bowled someone else out. I like that job – I weed the garden, and when they shout, 'Oi! Mum!' I yell, 'Woohoo! Yeah!' and applaud wildly from whichever shrub I'm currently underneath. Sometimes I get absorbed in gardening and miss my cue, and then they throw the ball at me to focus my attention.

After tea Blake and I practised making an avocado parrot (his class are doing vegetable figures at the school flower show tomorrow). We mutilated two unripe avocados in our attempts, and he has another two, along with a sharp knife, a packet of toothpicks and a carrot for beak and feet, in his bag. It's a shocking waste of avocados – I wish we'd gone for a potato parrot. A secondary concern, which really should be the one foremost in my mind, is that Blake's knife control is pretty shaky. He may lose a finger.

Ellie's class are making flower arrangements in novelty containers. She has selected a sheep skull for a container, and picked a selection of magenta manuka, scarlet nasturtiums and bright orange English marigolds with which to adorn it. Personally, I'd have gone for a prettier pastel palette – creams and greens and soft peaches – but I expect she's right. If you're decorating a skull you might as well be garish.

Thursday 7 November

My goodness, I'm tired of Diane. We had to shift Christmas lunch to the twenty-second because she and Thomas are spending Christmas Day with her parents. Then we had to shift it again, to Christmas Eve dinner, so they could spend the weekend of the twenty-first and twenty-second at the beach. I'm working on Christmas Eve, which will make the glazing of hams and the roasting of chickens complicated, but that's okay; nothing else matters as long as Diane is happy. She's also in a snit about Thalia's wedding being held in our garden; *her* house is the family homestead. She doesn't want Thalia to be married at her place, but she doesn't want her to be married at my place either. And *also*, while I'm raking up grievances, this is the woman who gave me a pump bottle of moisturiser for my fortieth birthday (we gave her a fancy deckchair). In a burst of passive-aggressive vindictiveness, I gave the moisturiser to the kids to use on the piglets, whose skin was a little scaly at the time.

*

Blake got off the bus this afternoon and burst into tears – his avocado parrot was unplaced at the flower show. First place was taken by a pineapple owl. I mopped up his tears and, when he'd semi-recovered, delivered a very moral little speech about how of *course* it's disappointing not to win but you can be proud of yourself as long as you tried your best, and losing is terribly good for you. If you don't ever lose, you run the risk of becoming like Lucius White, who is both a sports superstar and an arrogant little tosser.

Ellie's floral sheep skull won first place, I think due to the originality of the concept. It was the outlier among a plethora of gumboot posies.

Great stress at bedtime – Pidge had flown high up into the big kowhai tree and wouldn't come down to be tucked into his box. Ellie the helicopter parent is not taking her child's increasing independence at all well.

Friday 8 November

In bed, after spending a happy hour squeezing blackberry thorns out of my knees and watching *Friends* reruns. *Friends* was my favourite TV program when I was seventeen, and I still think it's hilarious – that's a high bar. So many things I thought were wonderful at seventeen (long droopy beige jerseys, Ronan Keating, *Cosmopolitan* magazine …) have failed the test of time.

The blackberry thorns come from spending the morning crawling around on a riverbank with a pair of loppers, chopping down Japanese walnut and privet seedlings from between the baby native trees. James's cousin Nicola has managed to get all the local landowners and iwi on board, and extract the money for fencing off and planting 30 kilometres of river edge from the regional council. It's taken her years. The council were apathetic, some of the landowners were unenthusiastic and a few were hostile, a splinter group of the local iwi fell out with everyone else and blocked off the access ... I think I'd have given up in despair, but she's just quietly carried on, making alliances and joining committees and patiently wearing away the opposition. She is a heroine.

Having single-handedly organised all that fencing and planting, she is now single-handedly organising the weed control. A council-employed gang are contracted to do it, but council workers aren't known for their meticulous attention to detail, so she follows them to do the bits they didn't see or couldn't be bothered with.

There were five of us this morning. It was stinking hot, and that section of riverbank is all covered with old logs that you can't see until you fall over them in the long grass. There was a paper wasp nest on every second tree, and the spit beetles were approximately five centimetres apart. In four hours, we weeded about a kilometre of riverbank – one side, not both. Well, it's a start, and it's very satisfying to look back at the bit you've done.

Saturday 9 November, 8.15 a.m.
To do:

- Continue helping Nicola weed riverbanks
- Weed stream plantings at home (four kilometres of creek)

- Spray tradescantia (although probably futile – if there's a nuclear holocaust, tradescantia and cockroaches will be all that survive)
- Spray jasmine in bush below woolshed (about an acre)
- Check stoat traps fortnightly
- Dag ewes, mouth them, check feet and udders
- Finish PowerPoint presentation on managing drench resistance, to be delivered at a farmer discussion group next week
- Update annual animal health plans for farmers seen last week
- Find a workshop on Land Environment Plans, go to it and write ours
- Have garden looking amazing for February
- Write book

And instead of getting on with any of it, I am on a plane to Wellington to partake in a literary festival. *Why?*

Alright. I will now stop hyperventilating and pull myself together. It will be *fun*. It's not every day I get flown to Wellington and put up in a hotel; I might as well enjoy it. Mum's coming, and so is my friend Kelly.

10 p.m.
Met Kelly at the train station, and we shopped all morning. She bought a blazer; we both bought shampoo bars. Very environmentally friendly, although I fear the environmental saving in plastic shampoo bottles pales in comparison with the

environmental cost of my plane trip. We lunched with half-a-dozen literary types, all of them delightful except one who related a stream of anecdotes starring poet friends of hers I'd never heard of and killed all other conversation. Mum arrived in time for the high tea event. It went well, I think – people seemed to be laughing. We left feeling quite euphoric and made our way, via several very cool vintage clothes shops, to a fancy wine bar. We ordered wine and cheese, and felt hip and urban. Then we continued, weaving slightly, to a litcrawl event. Litcrawl consists of twenty or more events run in three time slots over four hours, in bars and galleries all over Wellington's CBD. The event we chose was packed, and the speakers were hilarious. We emerged feeling uplifted and invigorated and entertained, and found a food truck selling amazing Malaysian food. Hunger sated, eyes bright with anticipation, feeling hipper and more urban by the second, we continued to the next event.

We got there a bit late and stood at the back listening to a girl ranting about the patriarchy. She started with Joan of Arc and worked her way forwards through history. Her only comment appeared to be 'fuck you', which was tedious. Everyone else seemed to like it, though – every 'fuck you' was greeted with wild applause. Eventually she sat down, and someone else got up and started singing a song about menstruating. It was all so militant and over the top that I got the giggles.

I texted James to tell him about it. He sent back a picture of the kids (they were all out the back of the farm deerstalking), with the message, *Leave. Sounds very bad.* We already had – we went and had another drink. I suspect the crowd at that event would have taken his text as proof of the dismissal of justified feminist rage by a chauvinistic, insecure, controlling male.

My 'Women's Bodies: Conflict Zone' event was in the third and final time slot. The blurb was:

> *In 2019, women around the world experience compromised body autonomy: politics, parenting, illness, media … women's bodies are sites of conflict. Writers read from work that reflects themes of intrusion, battle and vulnerability but also strength, power and love.*

I was the last speaker, after a very moving poem about being a sex worker, another about the strains of being part Maori and part European, a beautifully written excerpt from a book that described a girl being beaten by her father and a poem about the trauma of having a caesarean. I don't think I fitted into the session very well but, anyway, this is what I said:

> *I have a confession to make.*
>
> *When I saw that there was an event in the Litcrawl program called 'Women's Bodies: Conflict Zone', about compromised body autonomy, I thought: That'll be women talking about how tough it is to be a woman and how it's just not fair.*
>
> *That approach irritates me; I thought I'd go to something else.*
>
> *And then I learned I was in it. Damn.*
>
> *The thing is, I don't want to deny for a moment that sexism is real, but I don't think that being a woman has*

been an obstacle for me. The attitude in my family when I was growing up was always: Of course girls can do anything – crack on. And we did. I'm a vet, and for at least the last twenty-five years there have been more girls than boys graduating from vet school, so the question of whether women can do the job as well as men is just sort of obsolete. Anyone who thinks women can't is so obviously a dinosaur that their opinion really doesn't matter.

So, I was thinking about that and feeling ashamed about my privileged life, and then I thought, Hey, isn't it actually worth celebrating? Things aren't perfect, but they're a lot better than they were for a lot of women. And it's a pity not to reflect on how far we've come as well as how far we still have to go. So – yay. Thank you, suffragettes. I'm grateful for the opportunities and the mostly level playing field that I've inherited, and I promise to make the most of them and not take them for granted.

Now that I've got that off my chest, I'm going to segue awkwardly into telling you about how my body literally has been a conflict zone (which I think is the reason I was included in this session).

I had breast cancer a couple of years ago. I found a lump and went to the doctor, who said, 'Probably nothing, but we'll check it out.' And after checking it out they decided it wasn't nothing, it was a nasty ductal carcinoma that had already spread to the surrounding lymph nodes, and we'd want to get right on to it.

I had five months of chemo – hair fell out, stomach lining fell off, didn't have enough energy to walk to the mailbox –

and then a mastectomy and all the lymph nodes to my right arm removed. They did a breast reconstruction at the same time – they took the spare fat from around my middle (which I thought was a bloody marvellous idea) and moved it to the chest. It was a twenty-hour surgery, and it didn't work; the blood vessels kept clotting where they joined them, probably because I'd just had all that chemo. They had to remove the breast again a couple of days later. And then, when that had healed up a bit, I had five weeks of daily radiotherapy. All in all, it was a fairly grim year.

Anyway, it worked, and I'm now cancer-free. And I'm so, so grateful. But I'm a bit of mess without my clothes on. I'm missing a breast, and the other one has an ugly purple scar on it where a very junior surgeon removed my portacath. It looks like she used her teeth, bless her. I've got a scar right across my abdomen, and it's all puckered at the ends so I have this permanent muffin top effect. The other fun thing that you might not know about having a tummy tuck is that they take out this big wedge of skin and then haul the bottom of the wound up to close the hole, so you end up with pubic hair coming up to your waist. Super attractive.

Anyway, sometimes I look at myself in the mirror and it gives me a bit of a shock. And then I think, How dare you grizzle about a few scars when you're alive, and there's no reason you won't live to ninety, and you can still do all the things you used to be able to (except swan dives in Pilates; not enough stretch left), and you get to see your children grow up. Get over yourself.

So I do.

Sunday 10 November

Mum and I met Kelly for breakfast. We perused the literary festival program and debated going to a couple of events before deciding that, actually, perhaps we'd just shop. Mum the Style Queen raised our credibility greatly – whereas Kelly and I get dismissive glances from fancy shop assistants, they rush up to Mum and say, 'Excuse me, but *where* did you get that gorgeous coat?' I bought a great dress (flattering *and* comfortable); Mum bought a ravishing linen top. Then Mum went to meet other friends for lunch, and Kelly and I retired to an extremely trendy cafe, where we drank artisan beetroot juice filled with antioxidants and vitamins. We felt so healthy and virtuous after the juice that we immediately ordered a big plate of hot chips and gravy.

The plane met a thunderstorm on the way home, which was exciting. I wondered whether death would be instantaneous when we hurtled into the ground, and pictured James and the children's grief. I decided that, while they'd be sad, the community outpouring of love and support would be a beautiful thing. I was just hoping that James's second wife would love the children and wondering if Ellie would think of me on her wedding day when we landed.

Monday 10 November

Very busy day at work. I got in at four from my all-day dog vaccination run, having done no paperwork and with half-a-dozen phone calls to return, to find Sophie heading out to put down an old farm dog. The dog's owner is a lovely man, and he had extended an invitation to any vet who had known and loved Milly to come out and say goodbye. I liked Milly, but decided my phone calls and paperwork were more important. Then, when Sophie had gone, I felt like a horrible person who has totally lost sight of what's important.

I finished my drench resistance PowerPoint presentation at 9.30 p.m. and tried it out on James, who approved. Whew. I should know it by now, but I'm always surprised when preparing a ten-minute informal talk takes about five hours.

Tuesday 11 November

I was called out of our pre-work vet meeting this morning to see a wounded baby mynah. It was limp and gasping, so I took it out the back, put it down on the floor and stood firmly on its skull. It seemed the quickest and most humane thing to do. I dropped it in the skip and came back through reception, where I unexpectedly met the man who'd brought it in. He asked me anxiously how the bird was. I said that I was very sorry, but the bird was badly injured and I'd put it to sleep. Well, he said, smiling bravely, at least the poor thing had a peaceful death.

Ye-es, but perhaps not the peaceful death he had in mind.

When I got to the woolshed where I was giving my drench resistance presentation, the day's program on the projector said I was going to be speaking for an hour. Someone else kindly took up most of my hour for me: a farmer who's also a big wheel with Beef + Lamb. I've heard him speak before and came away with the feeling that he thinks vets are harmless at best and shameless pedlars of unnecessary drugs at worst. But his topic today was the trade delegation he's just accompanied to Europe. There he breakfasted with various important people and gathered all sorts of vital information about markets and projections. I always feel like I should know more about the international trade situation than I do, so I listened carefully. But somehow my brain doesn't retain that sort of stuff, and the only thing I can now remember is that we must be careful to say Asian Swine Fever rather than Asian Swine Flu, lest the word 'flu' unleash a panic among people who think they'll catch it themselves.

My drench resistance talk went alright, I think – nobody went to sleep and they asked some questions. Then they fed me a very good hamburger, and I continued on my round of calls.

The last visit of the day was to vaccinate half-a-dozen farm dogs. After I'd finished and was packing up my vaccine, the farmer told me various interesting things. They were, as far as I remember:

- The spot where we were standing was, when he was a little boy, a mere kahikatea swamp, only good for housing a few endangered bitterns. And now look at it. (I looked. It is now a thistly, swampy, impoverished paddock.)
- The new legislation that provides funding for fencing off land and planting trees is stupid and will accomplish nothing of any use at all. It is also an insult to the hard work of the men, including his father, who cut the bush down in the first place.

- You used to be kept awake at night around here by the kiwis calling in the hills. The kiwis have gone now; it's a bit of a shame, but nothing can be done about it. There's no point in even trying to thin out the wild pigs and cats and stoats that killed them all.
- Even if you could get rid of rats, you shouldn't. They're a vital component of the New Zealand ecosystem – they pollinate various native flowers and fruits. (??!!!) Some of those native fruits are delicious and he used to eat quantities of them as a child, although there are none left now.

This Caretaker of the Land had white tidemarks at the corners of his mouth and a nose drip. I'd been quite cheerful before our chat, but I drove back to the clinic in a deep gloom.

Wednesday 13 November

I had a last-minute-notice appointment at the breast care centre today to ultrasound the little lump in my armpit. You hear a lot about the inadequacies of the public health system, but I think it's awesome. One week from referral to appointment. Legends.

The breast care centre is wonderful, but I think the hospital parking building was probably designed by Crowley from *Good Omens*. (That's the coolest premise; in the old days, demons used to tempt and corrupt people one soul at a time, but Crowley realised that it's much, much more practical and efficient to do Satan's work by tarnishing a large number of souls just a little bit. Telemarketing, traffic jams, meaningless bureaucracy,

HR departments ... all evidence of Crowley's evil genius. It makes such good sense that if it isn't true, it should be.) I know the hospital parking building well, so I built in an extra half-hour to navigate it. I was still late to my appointment. I encountered several anxious, elderly drivers who didn't know to take the ramps between levels really wide and thus blocked all traffic in both directions, and finally found a car park on level fourteen. If that building isn't Crowley's magnum opus, it was designed by someone spectacularly cunning and nasty from the DHB's finance department, who hypothesised that if the stress of parking kills the sickest and feeblest visitors to the hospital before they make it inside, you don't have to squander valuable time and resources curing them.

I had my ultrasound – the diagnosis was scar tissue plus perfectly normal lymph node. Which was wonderful, but surprising, since I was told those lymph nodes had all been removed. Apparently, it's normal for them to miss a couple. I was a trifle disconcerted by that, when the whole point of having them taken out was that some were cancerous, but on the other hand, if I still have a lymph node, I'm surely less likely to get lymphoedema, which is incurable and causes your arm to puff up with fluid. To minimise your lymphoedema risk you just have to avoid cuts, burns and scratches to that arm for the rest of your life. Probably quite easy if you have an office job, no pets and no garden.

Thursday 14 November

Woke up feeling slightly jaded, after an interrupted night. One of the pet lambs had got through the fence into Dan's place and spent the night running up and down the fence line outside our bedroom, bleating. It was almost but not quite annoying enough to get up and do something about. At around two o' clock, James rolled over and muttered, 'I'm going to get up and shoot the little bastard,' but he fell asleep again before he could act on it.

I went out this morning to rescue the lamb. He was very relieved to see me, but wouldn't let me quite close enough to catch him. I sat down in the grass and looked non-threatening for a few minutes to lull him into a false sense of security, and then pounced. I missed, and he looked at me scornfully, trotted down the hill and slipped effortlessly back through the hole in the fence through which he'd escaped. Why the hell couldn't he have done that last night, if it was so easy?

In a burst of domesticity/writing avoidance, I washed the car this morning. Pidge was entranced – he sat on my head cooing excitedly while I hosed the soap off, and then flew down to drink from the puddles. The soapier the puddle the more he drank. He is a dark, metallic grey, with purple neck feathers and one tiny tuft of baby down left on the very top of his head, and he's finally grown into his beak. Bean the cat has lost interest in him now that he's not fluttering and crash-landing across the lawn in fits and starts, and has moved her attention to the family of baby rabbits in the orchard. Cats really don't grasp the concept of good sportsmanship.

Then I filled the backpack sprayer with a mixture of double-strength Roundup and single-strength Escort, which I hope will prove lethal to jasmine but not to me, and set off down into the bush below the house. It was very steep, and the jasmine stems hung down in curtains. I sprayed everything I could reach, but I couldn't get to the thickest stuff in the middle. Hopefully the edges I sprayed will die back, and then I'll be able to fight my way a bit further in. A few times I got hopelessly tangled up like a fly wrapped by a spider, and wondered how long I'd hang there before my family missed me and mounted a search operation.

Friday 15 November

Blake took on the role of my secretary this afternoon and answered a text message for me. A woman I don't know very well wanted to drop in and pick up a bag of grapefruits for marmalade – she doesn't have a tree, and I offered her some last week. 'Write: *Of course, if we're not home just help yourself*,' I instructed.

It was some time later when I looked at my phone, and discovered he had sent the message: *If were not there go for it* 💩 Blake has now been sacked as secretary.

Pidge didn't come home tonight. Ellie is taking it hard.

Saturday 16 November

The children are at an all-day dance concert rehearsal. It goes from ten till six. *Eight* hours! The concert is a huge undertaking – there are about fifteen classes, from preschoolers to adults, and they perform three dances each. They all change costumes between dances and do some of their dances in combination with other classes, and I am totally in awe of the woman who teaches them and organises the whole thing. All I have to do is find a few extra bits of costume, buy concert tickets for hapless relatives and get the children to the right place at the right time wearing the right clothes. That's almost too much for me; if I had to choreograph a 150-person, three-hour-long dance concert, choose the music, teach the 150 people their steps, decide what they should wear and procure it for them, my brain would melt and trickle out my ears. Oh, and she also writes every child a personalised certificate and performs a flawless solo dance of her own. And she's warm and radiant and slim and beautiful, with gorgeous hair and a perfectly flat stomach. Not that I'm jealous. Not at all.

The children had to be in their costumes for Dance One, with hair and makeup all done, when they arrived at the rehearsal. It took me half an hour and a serious amount of back-combing to do Ellie's hair according to the picture; it had a sort of central quiff and then rows of French plaits underneath. How James will manage to replicate it next weekend for the concert, when I'm away, I have no idea. Actually, that's not true; I know just what he'll do. He and the kids will arrive at the venue with Ellie's hair undone, he'll look helpless, and some capable woman will come forward and sort it out. I'm not disparaging him for a second; I use the exact same technique to get some nice man to back the trailer for me when I'm picking up farm supplies from town.

Amy, bless her, offered to take my children as well as hers to the rehearsal. We arrived at her house to find her frantically applying sparkly eyeshadow to her two little girls. 'We'll be late!' she cried despairingly. 'I forgot I had to make them look like prostitutes!'

Tuesday 19 November
Excellent joke Ellie brought home from school:

> Q: What's red and bad for your teeth?
> A: A brick.

Work was very quiet today. This gave me time to finish my overdue animal health plans, organise my inbox, book in my ute for panelbeating, read *Vetscript*, refresh my memory on the causes of abortion in sheep, look at plants and second-hand books on *Trade Me* and drink too much coffee. A veterinary Pilates session was considered, but by three we were all too apathetic to do it. I can totally see why people who have been on the dole for a while just slop around the house watching daytime TV – there's something so paralysing about having nothing urgent to do.

On the way home I listened to a podcast about how to go about being a writer, in case it was full of handy tips that would ignite my career. There was lots of stuff about the importance of building your social media presence, which I have heard many times before but ignore because I hate it so much. I know it's ridiculous, but the thought of putting something on Facebook fills me with terror and despair. What should I post? Look-at-my-charming-country-lifestyle pictures of flowers and pet lambs and nice green vistas? Win-a-copy-of-my-latest-book competitions? Inspirational quotes? There are people who do that stuff genuinely well, without being lame or needy or boring – but I'm not at all sure I could pull it off. I prefer being silent and mysterious. My chances of shooting to fame using this method are small, I admit, but it's much less stressful.

I was paying the bills tonight and James was filing them when we heard broken sobbing from down the hallway. We retrieved Blake and cuddled him, and eventually he stopped crying for long enough to tell us that he was sad because he was going to die, and we were going to die, and then we'd all just be gone. A long conversation followed, in which I offered the following consolations:

- Everyone dies, and their body breaks down – but then all their cells are part of everything else again, in a beautiful never-ending cycle. (*Northern Lights*)
- Nobody knows if your soul carries on somewhere after death, but wouldn't it be lovely if it did, and you found yourself somewhere like here, but better? (*Narnia*)
- Even if this life is all we get, and when we die we're gone forever, this is pretty good.
- You'll leave your mark on the world by leaving it better than it was when you arrived. (*Northern Lights* again, I think – building the republic of heaven where you are.)

My spiritual beliefs appear to be derived solely from children's books. Well, people base belief systems on sillier things.

Wednesday 20 November

Blake made himself a ham-and-lettuce sandwich for his school lunch this morning, carried it around the whole family to show it off and announced, 'This sandwich is a masterpiece of life.' I'm not sure what that means, but chose to take it as proof that he had recovered from his acute-onset existential dread.

When James and I went out to feed the dogs tonight, in the soft purple dusk, there was a deep, throbbing whir all around us caused by thousands and thousands of bronze beetles in flight. They've stripped every leaf off a cornus and two chestnuts that have done nothing to deserve such treatment, and are settling in a way that bodes no good all over the waxy cream-coloured trumpets of my super-special *Nuttallii stellata* rhododendron. I can't think of any way to remove them so am practising bronze beetle appreciation. Such pretty, shiny little creatures, with such a soothing hum. Maybe.

Friday 22 November

I'm at Clare's house in Whitford, tucked up in a very comfortable bed with crisp white sheets after a delightful evening of gossip and Thai food. It would be perfect, if only I wasn't racked with guilt.

When I left home this afternoon James had just rushed in, hot and sweaty from dagging the last mob of ewes, to take Blake to cricket in town and Ellie to the school disco. Then, in the morning, he has to get them both dressed and organised and provisioned for the dance concert, drop them off, come home to move stock and give two mobs of calves copper bullets and clean out the fertiliser bin, drive back into town, take the children out for dinner between shows and sit through three hours of concert.

In comparison, my agenda for tomorrow is something like:

Catch ferry to Waiheke Island
Brunch
Light shopping
Visit wineries
Sit on beach
Dinner in nice restaurant

James just sent me a text message reading: *Good night sweat pea*. (Spelling is not James's strong point.) Guilt swelling to epic proportions.

Sunday 24 November

We're sitting on a tiny little beach under a pohutukawa tree – at least I'm sitting; Clare and Suzanne are both asleep, Clare on her stomach and Suzanne on her back. Soon we'll have to get up and make our way down to the wharf to catch the ferry and go back to real life.

Clare and I caught the early ferry yesterday, and Suzanne, who arrived on Friday night, met us. Her brother's holiday house is a charming place on top of a hill, looking out over the sea. We wandered around the shops and went for a much longer walk around the coast than we expected, due to taking the wrong path. The walk was lovely, but Suzanne was wearing strappy sandals that nearly cut her toes off. Luckily, we found a winery before she was permanently crippled, and stayed for dinner. The food was lovely and the wine was amusingly bad, and we were joined by two charming Italian men. One of them conversed with Clare in a low voice, gazing soulfully into her eyes, while the other talked to Suzanne and me. (We suspect they drew straws and he lost.) Anyway, they were nice, and they drove us home after dinner, thus saving Suzanne's toes. Clare's new friend was very keen to come in and continue his charm offensive, but she felt she'd been charmed enough for one day.

This morning we got up late, had a leisurely breakfast and found ourselves this excellent beach. We've been talking and napping and swimming for the last few hours; topics covered include:

Pilates (excellent)
Shapewear (revolutionary)
Global warming (terrifying)
Charming Italian men (fun for a change, but not to be taken seriously)
How to recognise bad debtors (by the words 'I don't care what it costs'. Of course they don't; they have no intention of paying anyway)
Freezing your eggs (good idea)
The chances of Reese Witherspoon and Nicole Kidman wanting to make a movie of my latest book (extremely slim, sadly)

Monday 25 November

Slightly puzzling farm call today. I was checking rams (palpating testicles for lumps, looking in their mouths to make sure their teeth are good), and the farmer wouldn't let me mark the culls.

Me: This one's missing a couple of teeth. There's a can of spray paint on that post if you want to mark him.
Him: Mm.
Me (several rams later): This one's really thin, with a tooth missing.
Him: Yeah, we'll go through them later and drench the light ones.
Me (reflecting that drench doesn't actually regrow teeth): Why not put a dot on the dodgy ones, and just use them as back-up?
Him: (bland silence as he opened the gate and let them all run away)

Well, fair enough. They're his rams. But if he didn't want to identify the ones with health problems, why did he want me to come out and examine them? Like I said: puzzling.

I vaccinated his dogs while I was there. One had a very matted coat, and he asked me to cut the worst of the knots off with my cordless clippers. I may have got a trifle carried away – the dog now has a number one haircut on his back and sides, with long hair on his tummy, legs and tail. Turns out a mullet doesn't look any better on a dog than it does on a person.

James found the August and September invoice for grazing Dan's heifers in the fruit bowl this evening. 'Oh,' he said vaguely, 'there it is. I thought it was in the car.'

'Shall I deliver it?' I asked. It is, after all, quite nice to get paid.

'No,' he said, dropping it back into the fruit bowl. 'I'll get right on to it.'

I think perhaps I'll put that invoice in Dan's mailbox the next time I go down the road.

As part of tonight's bed-avoidance strategy, Blake returned to the subject of death. Is Sir David Attenborough very old? Will he probably die soon? That will be a sad day, won't it? Will the Queen go to his funeral? Can we?

Tuesday 26 November

I've just sent a half-completed manuscript to my publisher to see what he thinks. I decided, after a few weeks' internal debate, that it would be better to check that what I'm doing is vaguely in line with expectations than to blunder on in ignorance and hope. Waiting for feedback is always nerve-racking. I read a Facebook post by another author recently that described it perfectly as a strange, Schrödinger's cat-type twilight zone, where you could be the most gifted writer of your generation or you could be a pathetic try-hard, and until you hear back you're somehow both at the same time …

Wednesday 27 November

We have a foster kitten. Just for a week, while the lady who's bringing it up is away. Ellie has assumed command of its schedule, and is currently instructing Amy's little girls, who I picked up from the bus this afternoon, in correct kitten handling. She's being very patronising, but luckily they don't seem to have noticed.

Amy's children are delightful. The older one talks all the time without stopping, loses things constantly and can't keep her clothes clean for five minutes; the younger one is systematic and meticulous, wants to be a scientist, loves dismembering dead sheep and is permanently hungry. She appears beside me every five minutes, gazes at me with enormous, pleading, china-blue eyes and says, 'Can I please have some *food*?'

When I point out that she's just eaten four biscuits and a banana, or three mandarins and half a chocolate cake, or whatever it is, she sucks in her cheeks and widens her eyes until she looks like an ad for a World Vision appeal, and stands in a corner of the kitchen, the epitome of mute suffering. It's very impressive.

I just noticed a bird drinking nectar in the grevillea. I looked at it idly to see whether it was a tui or a bellbird, and it was a sparrow. Since when are sparrows nectar feeders?

Thursday 28 November

We – James and Thomas and I – spent the day in the middle yards, weighing lambs, marking and dagging big ones to go to the works, vaccinating little ones and condition-scoring ewes. I feel pleasantly virtuous, and I hurt all over.

It was cloudy, but one of those still, hazy cloudy days that's hotter than sunshine. We ran the ewes and lambs up the race, and James marked fat and thin ewes to be either fed up or dieted after weaning next week. He let them out a side gate, and I pushed the lambs up onto the scales, where Thomas caught them in the combi-clamp. If they were over 35 kilos he dagged them and I striped them with blue chalk; if they were under 35 I vaccinated them, and then Thomas let them go and they rejoined the mob.

It was a good system – we had the division of labour right, so that nobody had to wait for anyone else – but my goodness, it was heavy work. The lambs were big and rough and jumpy, and some of them turned around in the race and had to be manhandled kicking and screaming up the ramp. I bought a tennis-elbow strap last week in anticipation of this very job, but left it at home on the bookcase. As James pointed out, this was a good way of keeping it clean.

Anyway, with lamb prices this year I can probably buy myself a brand-new titanium elbow. We marked over half of them to go the works, and lamb just now is *nine dollars a kilogram*! It's a novel and most exciting experience to be making money sheep farming.

On the way home to meet the school bus I met Dan, on his way to mow silage. We discussed the likelihood of a thunderstorm, and he said he'd decided to take one for the team. It's a well-known fact that cutting silage is even better than planning a barbecue or washing blankets for attracting rain clouds.

Friday 29 November

There was fifteen mil of rain overnight, and when I got up I found a text from Dan reading: *You're welcome.*

I did some writing in the morning and then went to the furthest corner of the farm to spray blackberry in the fenced-off area alongside the creek. It was very beautiful, and very quiet, and I was enjoying the sensation of being completely alone in a fresh and sparkling world when suddenly a deer barked, and there was a crack of branches in the trees across the creek.

I know perfectly well that deer are quiet and shy, and that the stags are in velvet at the moment, and that the chances of being attacked and trampled to death, even if I actually stood on a fawn, are practically non-existent – but none of those facts helped at all. I sprayed for another hour with a prickly, uncomfortable feeling between my shoulder blades, twitching at every rustle or flicker of movement, completely oblivious to the beauty of baby ferns and foxgloves and dew-starred grasses nodding above crystal water, then scurried thankfully home again.

James had come in early for lunch, and he met me at the door with the words, 'I didn't used to like mustard. But now I do.' I suggested I'd heard more exciting stories, and he squirted me in the face with a drink bottle. I tackled him, but was overpowered due to his superior height and ungentlemanly behaviour. We then had to assure the rural delivery lady, who arrived just then with a parcel, that we were only being silly and I wasn't the victim of domestic abuse. Very embarrassing.

In the afternoon I went down to school to watch assembly. Both children got certificates: Ellie for Caring; Blake for Communicating. What little angels. I welled up a bit as we were singing the national anthem, and actually shed a tear watching the new entrants class dance to 'Fight Song'. Most of them had no idea what they were doing, but one tiny girl in the front row danced flawlessly and with fierce concentration, like a miniature warrior princess.

I was surreptitiously wiping my eyes when the woman beside me whispered, 'Are you okay?' I explained it was only that the little kids were so sweet, and she looked at me pityingly. Then the man on her other side said, 'I cry at that shit too. And ads on TV.' I think that's awesome.

Checking on the kids on the way to bed this evening, I found this sign on Ellie's door:

> *Rules:*
> *No one is allowed to go in my room without me being there or I have to tell them too.*
> *No being stupid about any thing.*
> *No little annoying children i.e. Blake, Keagan.*
> *You aren't allowed to talk about stupid stuff or I will kick you out (litterally).*
> *You must read and respect all rules unless I say.*
> *No Blakes (unless I say).*
> *If I say leave me alone,* **leave me alone!**

I am underwhelmed by this example of Caring.

Saturday 30 November

Rushed down to Amy's to borrow high, sparkly shoes to go with my plain black dress, thereby lifting my work Christmas party outfit from the mundane to the unbelievably stylish. Or so I hope. Dan had put his heifers on the driveway (which is actually his land; we just have right-of-way), and as I leapt out of the car to close the gate I managed to smear cow shit on Amy's beautiful shoe and up the back of my leg. Glamour is very uphill work around here.

The Christmas party was great, despite our extreme reluctance to go. Lovely food, good conversation, pleasant company ... But it's hard to feel excited about late nights when you've been getting up before 5 a.m. for a week to manhandle sheep.

Summer

Summer is such a lovely time of year. If only things were a little better organised and we actually had time to enjoy it.

Ideally, I'd like to spend large chunks of summer lying under a tree on a nice grassy riverbank with a good book and a constant supply of freshly picked peaches and plums and raspberries and blackberries (the blackberries must be carefully checked for shield beetles, because eating a shield beetle is almost as unpleasant for the eater as for the beetle). I'd also like to devote significant time to going to the beach, camping, seeing friends and building precious memories with the children.

But summer is the season of hot, hard, serious sheep work – weaning and drenching and dipping and dagging and shearing and drafting fat lambs to go to the works. It's the busiest time for large-animal vets, too, pregnancy-testing cows.

An awful lot of those precious family memories end up involving sheep yards.

Sunday 1 December

I went up to Val's after breakfast to retrieve the kids (and the kitten), who spent last night at her place while James and I partied. She ran this year's Christmas dinner menu past me to see what I thought:

> *Homemade ciabatta with cheeses (including Val's amazing baked feta and her camembert topped with toffee, nuts and dried apricots) to start*
> *Baked glazed ham with mustard sauce*
> *Roast beef fillet with savoury butter (Val's savoury butter is so salty and tangy and delicious that I could happily eat it by itself)*
> *Roast stuffed chicken and gravy*
> *Roast vegetable salad with feta and cashews*
> *Green salad (sounds alarmingly healthy, but the lettuce is really just a vehicle for camembert and avocado and bacon bits and fresh snow peas)*
> *Crispy duck-fat roast potatoes*
> *Cherry trifle*
> *Chocolate pavlova roll with chocolate mousse*

Lemon cheesecake
Fresh strawberries and blueberries
Gingernut ice cream

Oh my.

Blake is apparently still much preoccupied with death; he asked Val and Trevor some searching questions about their ages and current physical health last night, and calculated that, as long as he's married by the time he's twenty-eight, there's a good chance they'll make it to his wedding. So that's a relief.

As we were leaving Val asked if I had a lot of rhodohypoxis this year (rhodohypoxis are tiny, lovely, star-shaped, summer-flowering bulbs, pink and crimson and white).

'Yes!' I said. 'I've got heaps; they're everywhere.'

Trevor, who had accompanied Val to the door to see us off, shook his head gravely. 'Have you tried a course of strong penicillin?' he asked.

I like that man more and more.

After lunch we dagged a mob of hoggets, supposedly dry but with twenty tiny lambs at foot. Docked lambs and all but soaked them in Cyrazin fly spray in an attempt to prevent the little dears from being eaten alive by greenfly. The job was supposed to take an hour, but the hoggets were large and grubby and obstreperous, and it took three. Temporarily very sick of farming by the time we'd finished.

Tuesday 3 December

Even more sick of farming. Got home from work and Pilates at seven last night, hunted in vain for nice things to eat for dinner and settled yet again for toasted sandwiches, kissed my neglected children and went to the woolshed to help James draft lambs for the truck tomorrow. We drafted until nine, and James moved the ewes away in the dark. He had a sixteen-hour day with ten minutes off for lunch.

He got up at four thirty to muster and I got up at five, and we drafted the rest of the lambs. The stock truck arrived at five thirty, and we had 653 lambs loaded by 7 a.m. It went very smoothly, but taking all those puzzled babies off their mothers and sending them to slaughter is my absolute least favourite farming job. This year, due to the wild success of the ad lib lamb-feeding regime, there were half-a-dozen pet lambs among the doomed. One of them came up for a pat before walking onto the truck. I tell myself very firmly that animal welfare at the works is wonderful and they don't suffer (which is true; I did a fortnight's placement in a meatworks as a student, so I've seen it) but I still feel like a murderer.

I went to a meeting at school this evening to discuss senior camp, to which I have been bidden. I had hoped this was because of my sweet nature and all-round charm, but no. All the other parents going this year are fathers, and they wanted a token mum to deal with potential sanitary pad crises.

Wednesday 4 December

Email from publisher:

It's marvellous. I LOVE everything about it.

YES!!!

Thursday 5 December

James rang from the woolshed at 7.45 a.m. to say there was a juvenile kereru – a native wood pigeon – sitting under the bamboo hedge, which is not the behaviour of a normal, happy pigeon. So after dropping the kids at the bus I took a bath towel and went to the woolshed to investigate.

We managed to corner it and drop the towel over it quite easily, and I brought it home. It's very young – it has its adult feathers but its beak is still pale and soft – and very thin, but apart from a graze on its chest I can't find anything wrong with it. I gave it antibiotics and pain relief and water and a handful of defrosted peas, which it obediently swallowed when I poked them into its mouth. It is now in a box in our bedroom, recovering from the stress of being prodded and force-fed.

I really hope it's just weak from lack of food, and it will make a full recovery. Its timing is impeccable; Ellie is still mourning Pidge, who has taken up with a group of feral pigeons in Dan's hay barn and pretends he doesn't recognise us when we meet, and I had to take the foster kitten back to work yesterday. She'll be delighted to have something else to look after.

*

The kids and I rushed into town after school to borrow the big cage from work, so as to house the baby kereru in comfort, and to buy James a birthday present. We returned in triumph with the cage, a pair of nice shorts, a book on the Indian Mutiny, three Pixie Caramels, two bags of lollies and a hard-covered notebook. It's not James's birthday until tomorrow but we couldn't restrain ourselves and gave him his presents as soon as he got home. He loved them!

After the kids were in bed James and I watched *Gardener's World*, which he recorded for me a couple of weeks ago, thinking I might like it. I liked it so much that I made notes on my phone as I watched. Worn out by all this excitement, we were tucked up in bed by eight thirty. I think perhaps we'd better take up skydiving or impromptu public speaking or something else sufficiently terrifying to lift us out of our rut. At this rate, we'll be wearing matching cardigans and beige slip-on shoes by Christmas.

Friday 6 December

Our young pigeon was bright and bouncy this morning. Ellie and I fed it another dozen peas and I gave it more antibiotics and pain relief, and then Ellie carried it out onto the deck on her hand (it had got so tame in twenty-four hours that it was quite happy to be picked up), gave it a final stroke, and it flew away. It swooped off down over the lawn and up again to land high in an enormous poplar at the bottom of the hill. Hooray!

7.14 p.m.
Seething with rage. I've just spent three-quarters of an hour trying to cancel Blake's premium subscription to *Prodigy*, an online maths

game which promises perkily that *Learning math has never been more fun!* He was desperate to upgrade from the free game, so as to have cool magical pets and goodness knows what else, and I feebly signed him up for a trial month, since when he hasn't played the game at all. I had expected this, and wrote myself a reminder to cancel the subscription before we pay for another month.

That website was designed by a *pro*. The parent login is all but unlocatable, I couldn't remember my password (which was different to the one you use when logging in to play) when I *had* located it, and the automatic reset-your-password email arrived with nothing written on it. After much rage and frustration, I realised the email *wasn't* completely blank; you just had to scroll down two pages and then to the far right. An impressive attempt to prevent people from ever cancelling their subscriptions. You really do have to admire that sort of Machiavellian determination.

Saturday 7 December

Val took all four grandchildren to Hamilton this morning, armed with $50 apiece, to buy their own Christmas presents, go out for lunch and play in the playground at the Hamilton Gardens. I am speechless with admiration.

I spent the morning in the garden, tearing out things that are past their best and making enormous heaps of weeds all over the lawn. I love making weed piles – it looks so productive – but my enthusiasm for raking the piles up is always very low. I've left them in the meantime, hoping someone else will be seized with the urge to remove them. This has never, ever happened before, but you never know.

After lunch – because if we stopped doing things with sheep

too suddenly, we might get terrible withdrawals – James and I dagged the cull ewes ready to go to the works next week. I reflected, as I pushed fat, stubborn sheep up the race, on all the people (myself included) who say about sheep farming: 'Well, of course we're never going to get rich, but we love the lifestyle.' I've had two whole weekends away in the last month, so I can't complain, but James hasn't had a day off since May.

Val and the kids got home at four. They had a brilliant day. The girls all have lovely new clothes, and Blake saved his money but had a wonderful time ferrying his outfits of choice to their respective dressing rooms and giving his opinion on what suited them and what didn't.

We went out for James's birthday to the Indian restaurant. I love that place – the food's great, the staff are super friendly and they have a sign on the counter saying 'Voted Best Indian Restaurant in Town 2018!', which is especially charming because it's the *only* Indian restaurant in town.

On the way home James turned the radio right up, and he and the kids did a flawless rendition of 'Chop Suey!' by System of a Down, word perfect, at the top of their lungs, in three-part harmony, with synchronised head-banging and air guitar. Apparently they practise in the car on Tuesdays on the way to dance class. I had no idea.

Monday 9 December

Leaving this morning for an entire week of school camp. Filled with a sense of formless dread – which is ridiculous. It will be great. I hope.

Friday 13 December

Arrived back at school at 2 p.m. Entire class and all accompanying adults completely shattered. Camp was fantastic – the kids were good, the food was delicious, we walked and swam (in multiple rivers and the sea) and toured a goldmine and played spotlight and had water fights and built a driftwood fire (the parents had quite a lot more fun building that fire than the kids did) – but it's such a relief to be home. A week of spending the hours between 5.30 a.m. and 10.30 p.m. with a lot of pre-teens who, although they're perfectly polite, would really just like you to go away and stop cramping their giggling and flirting, is about enough.

The greatest strain, actually, came from being tasked with assisting Mrs Mason, teacher's aide, former cafe owner and all-round legend, in the kitchen. Mrs Mason adores cooking, and her food is quite rightly praised by all. She's absolutely lovely, but I found helping her a fine line to walk – to be there when needed but not be constantly underfoot; to wash up pots and chop onions but not step in and cook anything; to be just a little bit less busy than she was while pulling my weight. I spent the whole week teetering between feeling like a managing shrew and a lazy freeloader. Which was no doubt very good for me – I'm too used to being the one in charge.

Ellie had a wonderful time. When we got home she staggered inside, snarled at everyone, got told off, burst into tears, retreated to her bedroom in a huff and fell instantly asleep.

Saturday 14 December

I caught James in a moment of willingness to use the chainsaw after dinner (such moments are rare), and he cut back a whole thicket of tree lucerne that was suffocating a very nice nikau palm. The collateral damage was fairly light – two yellow lilies and one shrub, which will recover – and it looks miles better. James got quite enthused once he was going (this is always a risk with men holding chainsaws – they don't want to start, but once they're going, they want to cut down everything in sight) and was very keen to cut off half a flowering cherry that's starting to elbow the big kowhai tree in the ribs. I was quite keen too – but a wood pigeon who was eating the cherries sat on a branch just above our heads and looked at us with accusing eyes until we decided that the tree should stay until after cherry season.

I bought a mango while doing the grocery shopping, as a special treat – mangoes are my absolute favourite food. It was about as big as my head, fragrant and golden and perfectly ripe. I had a slice at lunchtime, which I halved with Ellie, and nobly saved the rest to share with James.

I was digging grass out from between the stones of my new path after tea when he wandered past and said, 'That mango tasted a bit funny. Starting to go a bit like turpentine.'

'I'll eat it,' I said. 'I thought it was perfect.'

'Oh no, I finished it,' he said, and continued on his merry way. Choked it down, no doubt. Bastard.

Sunday 15 December

Went out to get our Christmas tree – a six-foot tall, perfectly symmetrical seedling pine tree on the roadside just beside our mailbox that we've had earmarked for the job all year – and found only a stump. Someone else, it seems, had the same idea. We settled for half of a taller, lankier seedling pine with a double leader from further down the bank, and are now telling ourselves firmly that we *prefer* the naturalistic, imperfect look.

Things I need to do before Christmas:

- Buy presents for entire family (so far Ellie is getting colourful silicone smoothie straws and Blake is getting nothing at all)
- Plan menus for special Christmas morning breakfast and Boxing Day barbecue and buy all ingredients
- Make a double batch of gingerbread men, hippos, unicorns and dinosaurs, and decorate in suitably Christmas-y fashion
- Finish spraying tradescantia and crack willow along the creek banks (first overcoming unreasoning fear of being savaged by a deer)
- See *Frozen II* while it's still on at the cinema (Amy assures me it's the best movie of all time)
- Mow lawn
- Finish retaining wall, which I dismantled several weeks ago on the grounds that I'd never actually fix it unless I broke it properly
- Write chatty, delightful emails to overseas friends (*not* the 'This last year Blake has made the New Zealand Under 9 cricket team, Ellie is making great strides with her swimming and conversational Italian, James won the Coast to

Coast and my latest book topped the *New York Times* bestseller list for seventeen weeks running' sort)
- Alter my cream lace dress so it looks more like a dress and less like a tent made out of Grandma's tablecloth
- Wash couch covers and cushions

With all this in mind, I just spent an hour making a tiny paper castle to hang on the Christmas tree. Perhaps not the most efficient use of my time.

Monday 16 December

I've just struggled out of bed (it's 6 a.m.) to escape from a tangled and exceedingly nasty dream. It was full of hiding without hope in a town full of hostile, dough-faced citizens, and being constantly found and chased and caught. There was a small child who kept being torn from my arms and marched off to slavery, and I was trying to catch a plane, and I had to catch a biting dog (James should have done it but he wouldn't, and I screamed at him for being a hopeless wimp). Then I found that the dog had the face of an incredibly ugly old woman with many chin hairs, and it wasn't aggressive after all, it was just a pathetic victim of the bad guy I was hiding from, and so I had to lug it with me up and down the stairs of an enormous office block (with no windows although it was on prime retail land on the edge of the sea, which for some reason seemed the final proof of just how heinous the bad guy was), thus completely spoiling my already slim chances of getting away. And Melissa had hidden a whole lot of secret papers in her sinuses (this made perfect sense at the time), and a guard was extracting them and I was begging him to be gentle and not hurt her, but he didn't listen and cut her face open with a craft knife.

The whole thing had a flavour of dull, hopeless panic. Yuck.

Blake has just set up the chess board and is asking me to play. He's not bad at chess – and he calls pawns 'prawns', which I find almost unbearably cute. In a year or two he won't be talking about the windscripers in the car, and asking me to inspect various bits of his anatomy to see if I can see any smudges (i.e. bruises). Neither will he cry, on learning that he can't come with Ellie and me because we're going to a ladies lunch, 'That's *racist*!' It's a melancholy thing, watching your children grow up. Which is a really stupid thing to say, if you spend half a second considering the alternative.

The most memorable call of the day was visiting a calf without an anus. The farmer called to offer us the marvellous educational experience of coming out and viewing this animal before he put it down, and he was so pleased at the thought that I agreed. I felt a bit peevish about it, since I really wanted to ring a list of farmers and book in their herd pregnancy-testing instead of traipsing around the countryside on a mission of higher learning, but Sophie and I went out to have a look.

We found a fat, happy, six-month-old calf that did indeed have no anus but was pooing with no signs of discomfort from a perfectly good fistula into the vulva. So we told him not to shoot her; she wasn't the animal you'd choose to become the nucleus of your breeding herd, but she would be delicious in another year or so.

'She needs a name,' he said.

I was struck by inspiration (a thing I only wish happened more often). 'Fanny!' I said, and we parted with expressions of mutual esteem.

Tuesday 17 December

Spent the day driving around at the coast in heavy rain, palpating rams. The rain is very welcome (although on balance I think I prefer watching heavy rain through the window to working in it) as we were 300 mil short of our yearly average. I know this sort of statistic due to being married to a Rain Geek who has recorded rainfall every day for the last ten years. I had a lovely day; all the farmers I saw were in top form, what with the weather and the unbelievably good lamb prices, and when the sun came out the raindrops sparkled on every manuka flower and grass seed head. Gorgeous.

Ellie has just asked her brother to look at an actor in the movie she's watching and confirm that it's the same man out of *The Lord of the Rings* who went with Frodo all the way to the end and then turned out to be the king. The actor *was* Viggo Mortensen (Aragorn), and Blake is now explaining to her, with a wealth of detail, that he actually *didn't* go all the way to the end with Frodo; he ended up pursuing a band of orcs that had kidnapped Merry and Pippin. Ellie doesn't care at all, and doesn't like *LOTR* anyway, and just wants to watch her movie, but that is in no way discouraging him from putting her straight. Most amusing to watch mansplaining in action.

Thursday 19 December

Last day of school today! I picked up the kids from school (I was late, and had to park dramatically in front of the bus as the driver tried to pull out) and we went to the movies to watch the famous *Frozen II*. Very cool. Light on storyline, perhaps (now that's an ironic criticism coming from me, who can't write clever plots to save myself), but full of nice bits. I liked Kristoff's boy-band-style ballad, and whoever drew the water horse is a genius.

The movie theatre has a strict dress code, which I'd approve of if we ever managed to conform to it; I think it's nice that going to the movies is still a special occasion, and that the theatres are swathed in velvet with marble busts in the corners. But we had, as usual, forgotten footwear – Ellie's sneakers were floating around in the car boot, but we had to rush into Wrightson's to buy a pair of jandals for Blake. According to the definition of child poverty that looks at how many pairs of shoes a child has, we're really bad parents.

Must go Christmas shopping tomorrow. I'm not very good at it, probably because I always leave it till the last minute – but at least I'm better than my grandmother was.

My grandma was a lovely, lovely person. She was warm and funny and sweet, and everyone loved her, but she bought dreadful presents. Her worst mistake, she once told me, was the Knicker Debacle. She had a wonderful idea: she would buy nice knickers for all her nieces and sisters-in-law. Simple, cheap, pretty – it was a flawless plan. So, she bought everyone lacy panties in a variety of pastel colours, until she got to Aunty Annie. Aunty Annie was as wide as she was tall, and knickers made of ribbons and lace obviously weren't going to be man enough for the job, so Grandma bought her a pair of sensible flesh-coloured pants in heavy-duty fabric, reaching from waist to mid-thigh. And it didn't occur to her that this might possibly be insulting until the moment when the whole extended family were opening their presents after lunch and showing off what they'd got.

It was after this awful experience that Grandma's Undie Law was born. Never, ever buy any woman a pair of knickers larger than a size 12. If you know her bottom is bigger than that, buy her a size 12 anyway, and put in the receipt so she can exchange them herself. (Conversely, for men you must never buy undies smaller than a size L. Not even – in fact, *especially* not – for a man with legs like pipe cleaners.)

Friday 20 December

Realised suddenly this morning that the bills were due. The house, which I'm pretty sure I spent all of yesterday cleaning, looked like a bomb had hit it, and it was pouring with rain. Instead of rushing down the farm James lingered at home, play-fighting with the kids. And instead of being pleased that he was taking it easy for once, I felt cross and put upon and like the only person in the world who ever did any work.

I was paying the bills and snarling at Blake, who was helping me to concentrate by reading aloud to me, when Diane called. During the course of our conversation she noted that:

- *She* paid the bills on Wednesday.
- She sent all her Christmas cards last week. (I haven't written a single one.)
- How would I feel about starting Christmas Eve dinner early, with champagne cocktails and nibbly bits from four? Oh, you're working until five? Well, we'll start, and you can just catch up when you get here.

None of which improved my temper at all.

I'd more or less recovered by the time we went down to school prizegiving at eleven. The hall was packed, and it all went well. The chairman of the board of trustees, a very nice, very quiet man who hates public speaking, gave an excellent speech, and the leaving year eight kids spoke beautifully. (Also briefly, thank God – one dreadful year there were about ten of them, and they all spoke, individually and at length, about How Primary School Has Shaped Them for the Future. It went on for *hours*.)

Lots of certificates and trophies were given to lots of happy kids – and the final cup, awarded to the student who earned the most values tickets throughout the year (tickets are a serious business at school, awarded for Caring, Challenge, Communicating, Creativity and Contributing and kept track of via a spreadsheet system that seems only marginally less complex than the Nikkei Index), went to Ellie! She was so proud of herself. And so were we.

Saturday 21 December

The day started well, with James sending me a picture of a dead rat lying in a little pool of blood beneath a Goodnature trap (they put their heads up into a little cup to get the lure and trigger a gas-powered spike that punches through the back of the head into the brain; very quick, very humane). I was struck by the sudden urge to post the photo to Facebook, captioned *YES!*, but decided that perhaps breaking months of online silence with a dead rat mightn't be the best PR.

While waiting this morning for Ellie's best friend's mother to arrive and deliver Ellie's best friend, I started on the bit of retaining wall I dismantled a few weeks ago and have been plaintively asking James to help me with, to no avail. He came home for lunch while I was digging a (crooked) post hole, seized the spade from my hand and planted all four posts in about twenty minutes. I hovered, holding the level and ramming dirt and doing a little internal dance of rejoicing. Then he suggested a celebratory beer, so we had one, sitting on a sunny bit of wall. Marvellous.

Less marvellous are our weaned lambs. Two weeks ago they were growing like weeds – now, despite being vaccinated, they have something that seems very like scabby mouth and have gone from looking plump and delicious to looking pretty bloody average. We ran them into the yards this afternoon, supposedly helped by Blake and his little friend Keagan (they actually just stood around in the way, practising their secret handshake), and gave the worst ones an injection of long-acting antibiotic. Scabby mouth is a virus, so I don't know how much use that will be, but it might help to treat any secondary bacterial infection. At least it makes us feel we're doing *something*.

9 p.m.

I just went down the hall to say goodnight to all the kids. The girls were quietly reading in bed, having done each other's hair into elaborate plaits so it's curly tomorrow. The boys were putting the finishing touches on the secret handshake, which now looks worryingly like the palm-to-palm dance scene out of *Dirty Dancing*. They called me in to show it off, and I nearly passed out. 'Oh, sorry, we farted,' they said as I reeled back, choking, into the hallway. I only hope they don't asphyxiate themselves before morning.

Monday 23 December

I had a trying consult this afternoon with a woman whose little dog has a sore back. It's a chronic issue and she's seen a specialist, who performed various diagnostic tests and concluded there was a problem in the spine itself – probably a narrowing of the vertebral canal putting pressure on a nerve. Further diagnosis would involve a CT scan, which costs a couple of thousand dollars, and, depending on findings, spinal surgery. This would be very expensive and mightn't work, and she doesn't want to go there.

Well, that's reasonable. But she spent twenty minutes telling me that it Wasn't Fair. She should have a firm diagnosis and a concrete, guaranteed prognosis. She shouldn't have to stop the dog jumping up – it had knee surgery several years ago and she had to restrict its exercise for months, and she's not going through that again. She used to have two dogs, and this one is lonely and bored since the other one died, but she doesn't want to get another dog. The dog is too fat, but she can't bear to cut down its food. The dog adores the water and swimming would be wonderful exercise, but it's too much of a hassle to take it with her when she goes to the beach. The dog is on the best pain relief available, but there should be something better.

Eventually she convinced herself that there was nothing she could do to improve her dog's quality of life. I vaccinated the poor animal, then she pressed my hand and told me she finally felt Heard, and left.

The next dog in the waiting room was seen by Melissa. Dog with weepy eyes. She looked at the eyes, told the man it was nothing to worry about, waved him goodbye and beat me back to the vet room.

I want to be like Melissa when I grow up.

Tuesday 24 December

Nice day at work – everyone was feeling cheerful and festive. At four the manager carried in a great pile of wine and chocolates given to the clinic by various drug reps, and we divided them up. I got home to find James assembling rice salad and the kids already at Val's, and we hastened up the road, laden with food and presents.

We were the last to arrive, and the others had already demolished the appetisers and sparkling wine – which was good, because it removed the need to restrain ourselves.

We opened presents before the main course, because the kids would have burst with excitement if we hadn't. We don't usually do gifts for adults (an excellent development – the loss of a couple of scent diffusers and pot plants is more than compensated for by not having to buy half-a-dozen extra presents), but Trevor had bought beautiful little precision-engineered toy gliders for everyone. He and Adam and Holly assembled them all, and we had glider races off the deck. Diane and James proved to be the expert pilots in the family – they had a glide-off, with Thomas measuring the distance to ensure fair play. Diane won, and she was so excited that she ran in circles, yelling, 'In your *face*, loser!' at James.

Everyone was laughing at her and with her, and it was all absolutely lovely – until Thalia, eyeing Trevor balefully, muttered into my ear, 'The bastard's still not coming to my wedding.'

Oh dear, oh dear.

Wednesday 25 December

It's been an excellent Christmas. We got home from Val's last night feeling a bit fraught, what with Thalia's declaration of war, got the kids to bed and sat up, yawning and drinking coffee, until they were deeply enough asleep to sneak in with presents from Santa. Ellie doesn't believe anymore, but Blake believes *implicitly*. Tiptoeing into his room, we found a tray holding a glass of milk, a handful of gummy bears, two gingerbread unicorns, two carrots and the following letter:

> *Dear Santa from Blake*
>   *Hi the milk cookies and lollies are for you*
>   *But the carrots are for the rain dear*

Thank you for giveing me the knife last year now do you no what i want now? I want a motor Bike But i no it is to Big so can you please give me some money towards the motor Bike?

I called you on the phone your number is 0800 22 22 22 Can you please write Back Love Blake. But if you don't have time to write it is okay.

from Blake

Write please

(Not wanting to linger too long and risk discovery, Santa merely replied with: *Thank you! Santa xxx*, removed about half of the food and slipped a twenty-dollar note beneath a carrot.)

We had such a nice, cruisy Christmas Day. Just us for breakfast, and Val and Trevor came down for lunch. We ate roast chicken and new potatoes and trifle and banoffee pie, and then, learning that Val had never seen it, we watched the *Vicar of Dibley* Christmas episode where she has to have lunch with every parishioner in turn, quite possibly the funniest TV program ever made.

Thursday 26 December 7.50 a.m.

Having a minor panic. A wave of non-specific guilt is breaking over my head, accompanied by the feeling that I have about twenty crucial jobs to do and only really want to go back to bed and read *The Starless Sea* (Christmas present to self). But perhaps the jobs will seem less intimidating if pinned down on paper. I love lists – they give you such a productive, efficient feeling, even though you haven't actually done anything yet.

To do:

1. Shovel half a cubic metre of gravel off the back of the ute so we can use it to go down to the river for a barbecue (fairly urgent – barbecue is at lunchtime)
2. Remove weed mountain from the spot where the gravel is going
3. Get the gas hot plate out of the shed, make sure it works and fetch the gas bottle from the woolshed (assuming it's at the woolshed and not in some other random location down the farm)
4. Make bread dough so we can have cheesy flatbread at the barbecue
5. Defrost two packets of sausages
6. Clean the house
7. Fold washing mountain
8. WRITE (progress currently very poor)
9. Collect a trailer of dirt to backfill the retaining wall, and spread it
10. Make garden absolutely stunning by 29 February
11. Check stoat traps
12. Finish spraying tradescantia
13. Mow lawn

Okay. The first five items are urgent; the rest can wait. The one responsible for the acute-onset guilt is the writing (I didn't realise that until I wrote it down), but I absolutely can *not* do it just now, so I'll have to get over myself.

Right. Get up, get dressed, find shovel. Now. Go on.

10.38 am

Progress update: Ute deck clear; weeds picked up; bread dough rising; sausages defrosting; dishwasher mid-cycle; washing folded and put away (by children, after throwing of medium-grade maternal tantrum); recycling sorted; pigs fed (on leftover banoffee pie – pigs *delighted*); pigs' water bucket cleaned and refilled; small spindly dahlia mulched; lemon drink concentrate made; insect repellent, sunscreen, togs and hats located; compost bucket emptied (releasing epic swarm of fruit flies) and scrubbed. Whew.

There's a car coming down the driveway – our friends must be here early.

10.53 p.m.

They weren't early – it was Thalia. In tears, having just had an almighty pitched battle with her mother.

'Why *should* I have him at my wedding? I don't know him from a bar of soap!' she cried.

'Because your mother loves him, and you love her?'

'Why should *I* have to compromise? It's *my* wedding! Why can't she show her love for *me* by spending *one day* without him?'

I tried to suggest that it would be far better to include Trevor, even if he's practically a stranger, than to hurt Val, but Thalia was having none of it. The wedding is Her Day – it's not unreasonable for her to want Just One Day, is it?

'Yes,' said James, who had arrived home mid-tirade.

Now she's barely talking to us, either. I don't understand it – Thalia's normally such a sweetheart, and it's so unlike her to overreact.

We've never had a family feud before (granted, I say bitchy things about Diane, but never to her face). I wish we weren't having one now.

On the bright side, the river barbecue was lovely. The friends who joined us are the rare type that consider your children an asset rather than a drawback to a gathering. (I don't expect such an attitude – in fact, I don't always share it myself – but it's most heart-warming.) We swam and fished and talked and ate too many buttered flatbreads straight off the fire, and then packed everyone onto the back of the ute and drove home through the dusty golden evening light. A perfect afternoon.

Friday 27 December

This morning James and Blake went out to move stock, and I took Ellie, who was drooping limply around the kitchen, down to the creek to cut down crack willow seedlings and paint the stumps with weed killer. She grumbled for ten minutes and then decided that a morning of paddling in a shallow creek with a nice pebbly bottom, all fringed with long grass and ferns and baby trees, was actually quite lovely.

We waged war on willows for a couple of hours, came home and had leftover trifle for lunch – an entirely pleasurable experience until I hit a random piece of ham. Very disconcerting.

In the afternoon, in a fever of domesticity, I borrowed Val's leaf blower and used it to clean the cobwebs off the garage walls and various debris from inside the car. It was *awesome*. I recently learnt about the wonders of leaf blowers from a friend, and I can't believe I've lived all my life up until now in ignorance. The car was particularly impressive – you simply remove all clothing, jandals, swimming togs and water bottles from the vehicle, open the doors, point the leaf blower and turn it on. It has changed my life. Vacuuming cars is for losers.

Saturday 28 December

Both children have friends staying, and the house is filled with the sound of childish chatter. Also childish argument – we seem to be having a girl–boy war, exacerbated by a vicious attack on the girls' Lego masterpiece. Ellie's friend kicked Blake hard enough to leave a bruise during the counteroffensive, which was understandable but a little excessive. The girls have just gone down the farm to build a hut in a chestnut tree in the Peach Tree Paddock (which contains no peach tree), and I'm hoping tensions will de-escalate while they're away.

One of our hoggets has got into Amy and Sean's orchard, and made friends with their pig. Amy is delighted – they couldn't get two piglets, and she hates having a lonely pig. The pig and the hogget sleep together, and when the pig is fed the sheep joins it at the trough. It's quite disturbing watching a sheep licking up leftover gravy – and come to think of it, I'm pretty sure that feeding ruminant protein to ruminants is how you get things like mad cow disease – but never mind.

Sunday 29 December

Fell upon the garden like a demented whirlwind – only two months to go until The Wedding. Inspired by an episode of

Gardener's World about correct pruning techniques, I pruned the grevillea, the big pieris, a magnolia, four rhododendrons, an azalea, a cornus, two camellias and a flowering cherry. The lawn is now entirely covered in branches, which I have, of course, left for another day to pick up.

Tuesday 31 December

Work began this morning with a flurry of walk-ins (a dog for a pre-mating blood test, two vaccinations, a vicious Bengal cat the approximate size of a puma that had, thank the lord, come to the wrong practice).

Then Melissa and I pregnancy-tested the first dairy herd of the season. The farmer had booked in his in-laws to help with the recording, and it all went smoothly, after a small incident at the start where he had to rescue his mother-in-law from an enormous pet goat that was holding her hostage against a gate. (I've had dealings with that goat in the past; it's about five foot high at the shoulder, it's built like a tank and it hates having its feet trimmed.)

I like scanning cows, although my enthusiasm wanes slightly as the season progresses, the temperature rises and my elbows get sorer. It's a hard enough job physically to make you feel you've done something, and you get a little buzz of satisfaction each time you find and measure a calf. At this time of year, they range in size from peanut to newborn kitten, and they wave their little legs at you when you prod them with the scanner probe.

In the afternoon I went out to castrate a couple of calves. A simple, routine job, but nothing about it went quite right.

'You're not going to knock them out?' the farmer asked as I followed the first one up the race.

'No, it's best not to knock them right out on such a hot afternoon; they'll overheat,' I said. After which I gave the calf a sniff of sedative, just to get him to stand still, and he buckled gently at the knees and fell deeply asleep.

I explained hurriedly that this didn't matter at *all*; he wouldn't overheat because I would wake him up again the second I'd finished. The calf had one testicle that hadn't descended properly, and of course now that he was lying down instead of standing up gravity was no longer on my side, and it vanished somewhere up into his groin. Getting it back down again took a lot of fiddling around, bent over at an angle guaranteed to cause maximum back strain, and then holding it still so I could make a cut over it and pop it out. It was like trying to pin down a small greased animal intent on escape. There was no room to work and I couldn't keep the surgical site as clean as I wanted to. The stump bled more than I liked. A blowfly took a passionate interest in my surgical technique.

The second calf also had one retained testicle – this one so far up I couldn't palpate it at all, even with him standing. I decided that the risk of opening him up and fishing around in his abdomen far exceeded the benefits of castration, and went away. Oh well, it could have been worse. At least both patients were still alive when I left.

It was a beautiful, calm evening, and the garden was full of tuis. I picked up a few branches while James and the kids practised golf swings, and when the kids had gone to bed we watched not one but two episodes of *Gardener's World*. Bed at ten. Such a nice contrast to various New Years in my teens that were spent with a large group of people I didn't know very well, drinking something I didn't much like, wondering what was wrong with me and why I wasn't having a wonderful time. You couldn't *pay* me to be eighteen again.

Wednesday 1 January

Amy just rang to say she was washing her pig (I'm unclear as to why, exactly – I must enquire further) and it ate the soap. Do I think it will be okay?

'Absolutely,' I said. 'It will be clean inside and out.' (I'm actually not entirely certain that the soap will cause no ill effects, but why worry her?)

Thursday 2 January

James has made a list of all the farm jobs he wants to do before shearing, calculated the time they will take versus the time available, and is now fencing in a state of grim panic. I took the kids down to the creek to cut and paste willow seedlings, and discovered another acre or so of tradescantia blanketing a previously delightful stretch of bank. I fetched the sprayer and sprayed for an hour and a half while the children got progressively more bored and cranky, then went home for lunch via the patch of jasmine I've been trying to kill.

Oh God. The ground is completely covered with crisscrossing jasmine stems and they're hanging in thick, twisted ropes from the trees. The leaves I've sprayed have browned off, but there are great mats of shiny green foliage in the canopy, where I can't reach, slowly choking the trees to death. Aaghhh!!!

Friday 3 January

Ellie went to Thomas and Diane's for the day, where she and Rachel are making a tree hut. Blake has decided that girls are poisonous and wouldn't go. 'I just want to be with *you*, Mum,' he said. The mother-and-son activities he deemed suitable included him watching me tidy his room, me watching him play computer games and me timing him as he ran races around the lawn. I rejected these options and took him out to check the stoat traps.

It didn't go well. He trailed along behind me asking when we could go home, and was only briefly cheered up when I burst a very rotten egg that I was trying to lever out of a trap, and we found that it was completely full of maggots. How did they get in? It looked like something out of a horror movie, and the smell was completely indescribable.

Soon after that, he sat down in the long grass, burst into tears and cried, 'I can't go on!'

'Why not?' I asked.

'My socks!'

I checked his socks and found that they were stiff with ripgut brome seeds. Ripgut brome (best name ever) is a small, soft, innocuous-looking grass with seeds like arrow heads that worm their way through any clothing to the victim's skin, in what I can only assume is a mission to burrow right on through and eventually reach the heart.

I pulled out a couple of thousand and we went home, where I put on a movie for him and headed back out to attack the jasmine. I spent an hour cutting and pasting ropes of stems that were heading up into the canopy – this will, by my rough calculations, decrease the size and vigour of the jasmine thicket by 0.001 percent.

A friend told me yesterday that, on New Year's Eve, she found an old box of fireworks in the garage. So she made hot chocolate – with homemade marshmallows – and popcorn, and she and her husband *woke up their four sleeping children* for an impromptu New Year's Eve fireworks party. They had a wonderful time. Would this friend have chosen futile weed control over the opportunity to build precious memories with her son? I think not.

Saturday 4 January

Mum and Dad are here. They came last night, in time for the big annual river barbecue today. James's parents started having a barbecue at New Year for their friends and relations about 30 years ago, and it's grown into a major event. Dozens of James's cousins (the district is filled with them), current and previous neighbours, the minister who married James's parents, Val's best friend from primary school, my parents, Thalia's first boyfriend's parents …

It was a particularly nice barbecue. Lovely food, lovely surroundings and lots of nice people to talk to. One of James's cousins has been camping at the river and feeding the eels, and about a dozen came up to the bank and twined themselves lovingly around people's gumboots. They were completely unfazed by twenty shrieking children wanting to pat them, and the boldest ones came right out of the water to see what was going on. I'd heard that eels only secrete slime when they're scared, and it's true – these ones were soft and velvety to touch. Eels are adorable. Who knew?

One set of family friends had come down from Auckland for the day, bearing bean salad and kombucha and cauliflower rice. They were charming people (note to self: must not automatically classify all people who think white bread is poisonous as idiots), but their little boy has never been out of town in his life. I took him upstream for a paddle, and he was most concerned that we might get lost in the 'forest', 50 metres from the campsite along a four-wheel-drive track. He was so frightened of touching a prickle that he stood still and sobbed, but when I explained that plants can't move, so all you have to do is go around them, he grew bold and intrepid. He jumped over a baby gorse bush and threw stones into the water and we examined a spider's maternity creche on the end of a grass stem, and he was so proud of himself and so excited by his adventures that he nearly popped.

We got home at nine, cold and tired and happy. My only sorrow is that my darling children put all the sofa cushions, their duvets and the pillows from all of our beds on the back of the ute while I was doing something else, and thus all of our soft furnishings have come home smeared with marshmallow, spotted with sausage grease and smelling like wood smoke.

Sunday 5 January

James went out at six this morning, and got in for lunch at three. He went back out again at three thirty, came in for dinner at seven, and went out for the last time at eight to take the scales around to the bottom yards. The grazing company rep is coming tomorrow to weigh ten mobs of dairy heifers, each of which must be mustered close to the yards. There was a major water leak, and James had to fix the fence around the quarry before letting the cattle into that paddock. (Teenage heifers enjoy nothing more than jostling each other at the tops of unfenced cliffs.)

Mum is very worried about James. He works too hard. It's not sustainable. Nobody can work all the time without burning out. It can't be good for our marriage, or our family life. What can be done? Couldn't I help him more? Couldn't we afford a worker? She and Dad aren't rich, heaven knows, but they could contribute something towards wages to prevent their only son-in-law dying young from overwork.

I worry about James too. He *does* work too hard – not all the time, but for significant chunks of the year. And I feel bad for not being more practical help. I can't drive the tractor and the dogs won't work for me – but that's feeble. I'm a reasonably intelligent adult. I could learn to drive the tractor, and I could get my own dog. I just don't want to. I don't *want* to spend my last scraps of unoccupied time farming; I want to be a writer. My nagging guilt at this selfishness is doubtless the reason I interpreted Mum's words to mean 'James works like a slave and you're a parasite'. I know that's not what she was saying, but I was so irritated I left her in charge of the kids and went out to vent my spite on the jasmine before I said something I'd regret.

Finally, success! I found a way to climb up into the canopy and get at the leaves of the bloody stuff, rather than scrabbling around on the ground among the stems. It was so thick I could walk around three metres above the ground on great green mats of foliage. I sprayed everything in sight – I felt like Rambo, machine-gunning swathes of enemies – and returned to the house glowing with satisfaction. (Also glowing with pink spray dye; there was a playful little breeze up in the treetops.)

While I was away Mum discovered a petrified rabbit beneath Ellie's bed. Not ideal, but it could have been worse. I think my ultimate housekeeping low, to date, was the day I smelt something nasty during a phone interview with an Australian newspaper, tracked the smell to its source and found a fly-blown sausage under the couch. Like, *seriously* fly-blown. *Seething.* I'm just glad we weren't doing the interview via Skype.

Monday 6 January

Mum and Dad have departed to tour the vineyards of the Wairarapa, bearing Val with them. They'll return on Sunday and will take Ellie and Blake back up north with them for a holiday at the beach. I'm so glad Val went – Mum's very good at listening and sympathising, and it will be nice for Val to have a break from wedding nastiness.

Thursday 9 January

I got an after-hours call at quarter past seven this morning to see a fitting calf. You don't often get morning calls at this time of year, and the kids and I were just on the way out to help James drench lambs. I rang him to postpone and rushed off to see the calf. I was met by an offhand woman who made it fairly obvious that she felt I could have tried harder and arrived earlier, so as not to make her late for work. I dragged the calf out of a barbary hedge (calf large, hedge prickly), gave it thiamine and anti-inflammatories, sedated it to stop the seizures and sat it up, while she stood by, metaphorically tapping her foot. Then she shooed me away and hurried off. I drove away in a medium-sized snit. It wasn't *my* fault her calf got sick. And I'd probably just saved its life. I diagnosed it at a glance, and treated it promptly and skilfully. With no help from her. At considerable personal inconvenience. Which was kind of awesome, considering that I'm *much* busier and more important than she is.

At which point I remembered that going to after-hours calls is part of my job, and that people who are paying for your services aren't actually obliged to fall to their knees in gratitude when you turn up and do what they're paying you for. Must watch the tendency to become precious and self-important. It's very uncool.

The lambs look really good. They've recovered beautifully from the hideous face infection – whether because of or in spite of the antibiotic I have no idea, but thank goodness. The middle yards aren't well designed for drenching (rebuilding them is on the five-year list and has been for ten years) – either you run them up the race in single file, which takes forever, or you hold them in the diamond-shaped pen leading into it. That's much quicker, but the diamond is just a trifle too wide for two people, so James and I drench with arms and legs spread starfish-style, in constant fear that we won't be able to hold them and there'll be a lamb tsunami, where the ones we haven't drenched yet surge past us to mingle with the ones we have.

It went well today. No tsunamis, and everyone kept their tempers. (This is always helped by having a non-family member along with us; this morning we had Holly, who arrived at breakfast time to consult with Blake about a science experiment which has so far required a litre of cooking oil and a box of urine alkalinising sachets.)

The shearing contractor rang last night – the shearers will start either Saturday or Sunday. Hallelujah. They'll be here for three full days, so that's three hot lunches, three morning teas and three afternoon teas for seven people – three shearers, two shed hands, one presser and James. Morning smoko is at nine, lunch at eleven thirty and afternoon smoko at two thirty. I don't know what would happen if the food was late, and I don't want to know. (Years ago, Val told me that the first time she fed the shearers she got confused and assumed lunch would be at noon. She didn't tell me what happened; she just went pale and trembly and I assumed the fallout was appallingly bad.) I won't be here on at least one and possibly two of the days because I'm working.

However, all things are possible with sufficient organisation. James can dash over from the shed to turn the oven on as long as I have everything else ready. Right, what to feed them?

Menu

Day 1
Morning smoko
 Sausage rolls
 Banana cake

Lunch
- *Lasagne*
- *Salad*
- *Homemade bread*

Afternoon smoko
- *Peanut brownies*
- *Ginger crunch*

Day 2

Morning smoko
- *Cinnamon buns*
- *Lemon cake*

Lunch
- *Shepherd's pie*
- *Coleslaw*
- *Homemade bread*

Afternoon smoko
- *Chocolate brownies*
- *Teacake*

Day 3

Morning smoko
- *Cheese scones*
- *Chocolate slice*

Lunch
- *Chicken pie*
- *Salad*
- *Homemade bread*

> *Afternoon smoko*
>   *Custard squares*
>   *Chocolate chip biscuits*
>
> *Also a massive thermos of cold lemon drink to be on tap at the shed.*

Friday 10 January

I made lemon drink concentrate, chicken pie, cinnamon buns and chocolate slice before being brought to a temporary standstill by lack of flour.

I was adding it to the shopping list when I found I'd written down 'mice'. *Why?* What should I have written instead, and will I remember in time? While pondering this question I noticed that I only shaved one leg in the shower last night. I think I might be losing my mind.

9.15 p.m.
I have it. *Mince*. Whew.

Saturday 11 January

The weather, which has been unseasonably chilly with howling winds, changed today to still and roasting. The shearers will be here tomorrow. We spent the morning finishing the dagging in the shadeless wasteland that is the middle yards. The kids were wonderful — at least, Ellie was entirely wonderful and Blake moderately so. They are both very pleased about the shearing tomorrow, and are planning to spend all day at the woolshed. Blake actually requested that we read early tonight so he could be asleep by seven thirty, in preparation for getting up at 6 a.m. to go with James. He's gone to sleep in his clothes to save time in the morning, and has borrowed my cell phone and set an alarm, just in case James doesn't wake him.

This afternoon I made lasagne, shepherd's pie, banana cake, salad and chocolate brownies. Now ready for anything.

James just got in – it's nine forty-five – after penning up the lambs for tomorrow.

Sunday 12 January

I'm feeling slightly crushed after one of the shed hands took a bite of lasagne at lunchtime, put down her fork and said, 'Got any sauce, miss?'

I brought her the tomato sauce, and first she, then most of the others, poured it copiously over their food. Evidently my lasagne was less succulent and delectable than I thought.

Well, pride goeth before a fall. For the last few years I've had a smug, comfortable sort of feeling about my cooking, dating from the time when I heard the presser saying to a shearer who'd never been here before, as they kicked off their shoes at the door, 'You get the *mean* feed here, bro.' (Maybe the nicest compliment I've ever had.)

It's always a bit of a strain when the shearers come over for lunch. They're always very quiet, and although I want to be friendly, I can never think of anything to say apart from, 'How's it going? Is it very hot in the shed?' I end up fiddling around in the kitchen, trying not to look like I'm hovering but wanting to be within earshot if they need anything (i.e. more sauce), while they bolt their food in near silence and leave as quickly as they can.

Derek is the sole exception. He's a lovely man, somewhere in his fifties, and he's a connoisseur of the arts. He assumes I am too, seeing as I write books, and he always asks what I think of various recent film festival movies and pieces of avant-garde interactive theatre, none of which I've ever even heard of. I always feel very humbled and parochial after talking to Derek, and vow to become better educated before I next see him, but I never do.

Monday 13 January

Mum and Dad arrived last night, after a delightful week in the Wairarapa. They're going to deliver the smoko to the shed this morning and then carry on north, taking Ellie and Blake with them. I'm so glad – we were feeling like horrible child-labour-exploiting parents.

Tuesday 14 January, 6.15 a.m.

Day three of shearing. We got twelve mil of rain last night that we weren't expecting but were very happy to see (James got *most* of the sheep into the shed before it started, and hopefully the rest will dry out during the day). I'm leaving at seven thirty this morning to get to our most distant dairy farm, where Melissa and I are scanning 600 cows. I'll put the scones for morning smoko into the oven as I leave, and James will come and get them at ten to eight. There's a chicken pie and a coleslaw in the fridge.

8.30 p.m.
They got all but 200 ewes shorn – the ones that got wet last night didn't dry out after all – but they'll come back and finish them off in an hour or two on Friday morning, so it doesn't matter. Whew. James is asleep on the couch, curled up like a little boy.

I'm feeling temporarily very tired of vet work – actually, of all work, veterinary or otherwise. My elbow hurts, and it's only the start of the scanning season. Melissa's little dog thinks she's pregnant, although she's not, and she's in a foul mood. She's picking fights with Jess's dog and the clinic cat – it's like having a small furry woman with appalling PMT in the building. A man brought in a cat with a very bad eye this afternoon, which it turns out was seen last week and inadequately treated at the time. The owner was not very pleased, understandably. I just got a slap-on-the-wrist email from the vet at the local meatworks about a cow she suggests I shouldn't have certified for transport. She had a cancerous growth below her lower left eyelid – I thought when I certified her that it looked irritating rather than painful, and that being trucked to the works wouldn't be a welfare concern, but the vet who saw her when she got there felt it would have been more appropriate to shoot the cow on farm. Certifying animals for transport is a stressful undertaking at the moment – the regulations have just been tightened up, but nobody's very sure what they've been tightened up to. We could just refuse to write certificates for anything that looked marginal – but that's not ideal either. If you write a certificate for a cow with some lesion, you know that within a week it will have been killed. If you don't, there's always the possibility that the farmer will just put it in a back paddock somewhere to see how it goes, and it might languish there for weeks or months.

And to top it all off, I'm on call again tonight, and I was just shutting down my computer at five when the Nisbets called to say their dog had something stuck in its mouth and needed seeing right away.

The Nisbets are a lovely family. Pillars of the community. But their dog is an aggressive, 54-kilogram Rottweiler that hates everyone in the whole world except them.

He arrived muzzled, but the muzzle was a flimsy plastic thing he could have got off any time he liked. I performed a thorough oral examination (i.e. peered at his mouth from five metres away), saw neither dribbling nor swelling, gave his owners an anti-inflammatory tablet to hide in his dinner and asked them to come back in the morning at nine thirty. There's a small chance that he'll miraculously recover overnight – and if not, at least tomorrow morning there'll be other people around at work to apply pressure to my femoral artery when he tries to rip my leg off.

Wednesday 15 January

Survived the Rottweiler. But what a performance. It took four people three goes to wedge him behind a door with a rope around his neck, pulled tight through the crack above the hinges, so I could jab him in the bum with sedative. (There was a low moment when he was all ready to go but I'd popped out of the room to consult with Jess about something else, and he tried quite hard to strangle himself before I came back. Oops.) But eventually we got it sorted and jabbed him, which made him sleepy enough to get a slug of ketamine into his vein. Finally, an hour after he arrived, I removed a sewing needle – still threaded – from his tongue. It took about two and a half seconds. If only we could have castrated him while he was asleep. Mr Nisbet agrees that's a good idea, but he couldn't quite bring himself to do it today. He'll book it in sometime soon – hopefully giving enough notice that I can invent some illness which will keep me home from work that day.

Just talked to the kids on the phone – they're having a wonderful time playing with Mum and Dad's neighbours' grandchildren. Mum and Dad's place backs onto the golf course, and they've collected over a hundred stray balls already. According to Ellie, Blake got one today that a man had just hit into the long grass. I suggested that harvesting golf balls that are actually in play would lead to nothing good, but I don't think she was listening.

Thursday 16 January

James and I went out after tea (tea was bread and butter with peanut brownies; standards have slipped without the kids home) to muster a little mob of ewes and lambs away from the woolshed. It was a gorgeous evening, with the hills standing up crisp and dark purple against an apricot sky, and the long grass all silvery in the dusk. Most beautiful of all was the mass of dying jasmine below us at the edge of the bush.

James went out ahead to open a gate, leaving me and Dream to keep the sheep walking the right way. As soon as James was out of sight, Dream sat down. The sheep reached the next gateway and stopped. I shouted to get them moving again, and

Dream just lay there, tongue lolling, as they surged back towards her. She continued to recline and smile as I screamed at her and ran back and forth like a crazy thing, and then, just as the mob broke and James reappeared over the brow of the hill, she got up and slipped smoothly back into action. Bitch. Anyway, *I'm James's favourite*, not her. I get to come in the house; she has to sleep in a kennel.

Friday 17 January

I have slumped. Today was the first day for weeks that I wasn't dashing around in circles trying to get things done, and instead of enjoying this unaccustomed leisure I'm as flat as a pancake.

Also, I'm on call this weekend, and my phone suddenly died this afternoon. Not for any good reason – I didn't drop it or get it wet; it just died. No response to charging, or to pressing and holding the right buttons. So I have James's phone, which is highly inconvenient for him, and anybody who tries to call or text me on my own number will no doubt assume I can't be bothered replying.

My glasses are so scratched that there's a blur in the middle of my field of vision – I rang the optometrist's, and they said to pop in so they could assess them, and I'd likely get replacement lenses free. So, after delivering the final morning smoko to the woolshed, where the shearers were finishing the last couple of hundred ewes, I went to the optometrist. It's a 45-minute drive, and I was nearly there when I realised that I was wearing my sunglasses, and that the glasses that needed replacing were at home on the kitchen bench.

*

Things looked up in the evening. We sat on the couch looking up old songs on YouTube (James had control of the laptop, which meant we listened to his choices in full and the first 30 seconds of mine) and eating plum and crème fraiche gourmet ice cream. Then I had a long, leisurely bath and read *The Grand Sophy* for the twenty-seventh time. Lovely.

Saturday 18 January

I had a call this afternoon to a cow that couldn't stand up; her left back leg wouldn't bear weight. She had a dislocated hip, and I was pretty sure she'd broken her hip joint at the same time – with a simple dislocation they're very lame, but they can almost always get to their feet. So we decided it would be best to put the cow down. At this point the farm worker whipped his phone out of his pocket and said, 'Can I video you doing it, just to prove to my friends that farming's not all happiness and light?'

For some reason – probably because I'm not very bright – I said doubtfully, 'Uh, I guess …' And so there now exists, somewhere on the internet, a video of me injecting pentobarbitone into the jugular vein of a cow, and then cutting open the muscles above her hip joint, post mortem, to make sure I'd got my diagnosis right.

When I told James about it, he looked at me with blank dismay and said, 'You idiot. I can't believe you said yes.'

Oh God. A group of lunatic-fringe animal activists will find the video, edit it and I will go viral as a hideous cow torturer, thus destroying both my career and the New Zealand dairy industry.

We're really missing the kids. Peace and quiet is overrated.

Monday 20 January

James met Dan on the road this afternoon, and Dan asked for his latest grazing invoice. I remember that invoice well. It was the one for December and January's heifer grazing, which James wrote after I reminded him several times. I put it in an envelope and slipped it into my diary to deliver on my way to work the next day. I don't remember delivering it, though. I must have lost it somewhere en route.

James has now written out a new one and made a great show of taking it to Dan *himself*, so I can't cock it up. I'm quite fond of James, but sometimes he's a patronising arse. (I pointed this out, and he put his nose in the air and said, 'I can be a patronising arse if I want. You're not the boss of me.' Patronising *and* deluded, apparently.)

I pulled off the road today to write myself a note about restocking my ute with eighteen-gauge needles, and saw a goldfinch stuffing its face on thistledown. It had its whole head buried in the fluff, and it was chomping away like the Cookie Monster. Very cute.

While not observing goldfinches, I listened to a great podcast all about mindful eating. Never diet, said the nutritionist who was being interviewed. It always fails; your body won't let you starve it, just like your lungs won't let you hold your breath indefinitely. You'll just set yourself up for a major blowout, and then a rebound surge of shame and guilt. What you actually need to do is listen to your body. If you're hungry, *eat*. But most of us eat when we're not hungry, and that's what we have to learn to recognise and combat.

It was a really good podcast. Inspirational, even. And yet I just finished all the rest of the gourmet ice cream, because it was there and it tasted nice. And now I feel sick. Oh well, I suppose at least I'm listening to my body now.

Tuesday 21 January

A long hot day that included, among other jobs, blood-testing rams with the aid of a bottom-patting farmer. I suppose one could be flattered at having one's bum fondled while wearing overalls and sweating profusely – but on the other hand the man's only criteria for female desirability is a pulse, so perhaps not.

At the supermarket this evening I ran into a very nice lady, a keen gardener who assured me loudly that she can give me gobs of poo. Gobs and *gobs*. A girl who was passing looked at us with horrified distaste – she may not know that Pooh is a very pretty collarette dahlia.

Latest news on the Wedding Front (sort of like the Western Front, except not so muddy and without – at this stage – any machine guns): Trevor may attend the reception but not the ceremony. Poor Thalia – she'll look back on this in years to come and wish that she could go back in time and give her younger self a good kicking for completely ruining her mother's enjoyment of her wedding. Or perhaps she won't. Perhaps it will crystallise in her memory with herself as the victim. Much more comfortable that way.

Wednesday 22 January

At work today I saw two lame bulls. The first one is almost certainly doomed – he had a fat foot, with pus in his fetlock joint when I popped a needle into it. I flushed the joint and put him on antibiotics and anti-inflammatories, but without much hope.

Bull two was even less successful. He was really lame – three-legged lame – and I couldn't find a single thing wrong with him, even after sedating him, scraping clean his hooves and palpating every joint from toe to shoulder. We finally sat him up again, and I made the really helpful diagnosis of, 'Well, either he'll improve, or he'll get worse and you'll have to shoot him.'

I left work a bit early and cleaned the house, fed the pigs, took the dogs for a walk, put in Bean's eyedrops, watered the plants, wrote detailed pet care instructions for Thomas, packed James's clothes and mine, took a shower and had everything ready in the car when James got home after moving and feeding out to every mob on the farm. Whew. We got away at four, as intended (a completely unprecedented occurrence), and bought ourselves Burger Fuel burgers, potentially the best takeaway on the planet, for dinner on the way. We got to Mum and Dad's place at nine and found the kids dancing up and down with excitement in the driveway. So, so good to see them.

Sunday 26 January

We had a gorgeous holiday. We swam and swam, sometimes by the pontoon in the estuary where there are rock pools and tiny foot-nibbling shrimp and a friendly baby octopus, and sometimes at the surf beach. The water was crystal clear and the waves a beautiful ice-blue. I saw a tiny, delicate, pure white seabird that I'm sure was a fairy tern. James slept for most of the first two days, and Dad and Blake and I went on an epic walk around the point on the rocks. It involved sneaking through private property (it's lucky James didn't come; he's far too law-abiding and won't do things like that) and slithering down dry hills all covered with nikau palm fronds. We met huge crabs, oyster beds, beaches with pink sand and beaches with tiny pale-grey pebbles and beaches with big round boulders perfect for rock-hopping. The others drove around to meet us on the far side, and we went out for a late lunch. It was all absolutely lovely.

We came home again this morning, and Blake met, for the first time, his *new motorbike*. (A year ago, James told him that if he saved $500 we'd pay the rest, and he got to $527 at Christmas. The bike was quite a lot more than $500, so the deal is that while Blake may call it his, he must let his sister ride it whenever she wants to.) Both kids were wildly excited, and they've spent the last two hours beetling around the lawn in first gear.

Monday 27 January

Today is a public holiday, and we all went out early to weigh lambs. The weather was quite cool and pleasant; the lambs were not. We drafted them into three lines – ewe lambs, wethers big enough to go to the works and tiddlers – and then drafted each line again, due to a percentage of obstreperous fence-jumping little mongrels. The kids were great, and we were all, miraculously, still friends by the end.

Then James carried on farming and the kids and I came home. After watching them ride the motorbike in circles on the lawn for an hour I decided I should really have another crack at the bloody tradescantia – I tried to sell them on the joys of coming too and paddling in the creek, but they've fallen for that in the past and flatly refused. So I went on my own. It was very hot, and I found another infested gully, but I've got used to that now and hardly cried at all. The trick is not to think about how big the job is, but just to go and do a little bit and then tell yourself it all helps. (Not a bad approach to life as a whole, come to think of it.)

After dinner we mounted an expedition to chase five lambs out of the neighbour's place. Thomas and Holly came to help us, due to the extreme wiliness and uncooperativeness of the lambs.

What a debacle. A semi-debacle, anyway; we did get three out of five. The last two evaded us. The dogs went the wrong way, causing James to roar at them and actually dance with rage, Ellie screeched at James not to be mean to the poor dogs, Thomas encountered a bull hole hidden in the long grass and fell off his motorbike …

After which we decided that 60 percent was pretty good, really. As we drove home up the hill in the dusk, I looked back and saw the last two lambs, drifting serenely across the hillside where they started, and I'm pretty sure I heard them sniggering.

Tuesday 28 January

I had a call today from a farmer who actually *wanted to sit down and go through her mating data*! This is incredible and unprecedented; we offer a free reproductive review after pregnancy testing as part of our value-added service, but very few people take up the offer, let alone *request* a meeting. The only issue is that this particular farmer had the opposition do the pregnancy testing because they were slightly cheaper. The logical thing to do would be to charge $200 for an hour of my time, but I'm sure she'd be deeply offended, and I'm too much of a wimp. So, no doubt, I'll do it for nothing and feel resentful. It's a terrible handicap, being a passive-aggressive people pleaser.

Sophie and I went out to pregnancy-test 90 heifers this afternoon, at a farm an hour's drive from the clinic. On arrival, we discovered that I had forgotten to bring a headset for one of the scanners, and that the second headset had a bent pin and wouldn't plug into the scanner. So we pregnancy-tested them all manually, one at a time up the race. Which wouldn't have been much of a problem, apart from being a bit slower, except that the farmer wanted them all aged.

I used to be pretty good at ageing pregnancies by palpating the size of the calf and the uterus, but now that we have ultrasound scanners, my manual skills are very rusty. If I'd been strictly truthful, I'd have said things like, 'Probably somewhere around nine weeks in calf, give or take a couple of weeks each way' – but a farmer paying for your services would be quite entitled to be annoyed at such vagueness, so

I said, 'Sixty-five days!' and felt guilty. (There was a dreadful moment when I said, 'Eighty-five plus days!' and the farmer said, 'Instead of seventy-five? That's the one you did already, that backed out.')

'I wish I was as accurate as you,' said Sophie as we left, rubbing salt into my self-inflicted wounds.

Assured her hastily that I am a complete fraud.

There are two flat stripes through two clumps of perennial phlox in the garden, where Blake and the motorbike have run amok. His confidence is growing faster than his skill. What with him and no rain for the last month, the garden is going to be a fairly average backdrop to Thalia's wedding ceremony.

Wednesday 29 January
IT'S RAINING!!!!!!

And … it's stopped. One and a half mil, according to the rain gauge. Hmm.

I'm reading the New Zealand Book of the Year. It's really good. Better (I admit grudgingly) than mine.

Thursday 30 January
The kids graduated to second gear on the motorbike today, and to the paddock below the house. Blake has taken to wearing his helmet everywhere – it's enormous and he's about two inches wide, so he looks like a lollipop. (James bought them each a proper motocross helmet yesterday, for over $200 each. I was appalled at the cost, and he was extremely self-

righteous about my selfishness in wanting to economise on the children's safety.)

While they buzzed up and down like wasps I cleaned the enormous cupboard in the hall – it had reached the stage where we could barely force the vacuum cleaner in, and to get things at the back we had to throw a child in over a wall of oil heaters, clothes racks and bits of dismantled electric piano. Very worthwhile job – I found a brand-new can of fly spray, several working vaccinating guns and a double blow-up mattress that Thomas and Diane might quite like back.

Friday 31 January

Ellie, Val and I went to Hamilton for a girls' day out – James and I felt Ellie was due for a treat, since the motorbike is officially Blake's.

Our first destination was Farmers, where, although there are many nice clothes, it's very difficult to find them in the maze of shiny white marble flooring and mirrored walls. You keep striking off in different directions, and finding that somehow all paths lead back to the same rack of mustard-coloured chiffon maxi-dresses. I keep meaning to buy one of those amazing steel-reinforced slips that give you a smooth hourglass shape beneath your clothes, but the effort of finding one in the identical mirrored aisles, and then finding the changing rooms, seemed so great that I feebly gave up and we retreated to a cafe for cold drinks.

From Farmers we headed to the city centre, where we drove in circles around a parking building for some time, first looking for a park (the sign outside said there were fifteen spaces, but they were all occupied by bastards taking up two spots each) and then trying to leave the horrible place without denting the car. Eventually we parked on the street, miles from where we wanted to be, and walked.

We lunched at a trendy, delicious *and* cheap Vietnamese cafe overlooking the river, which cheered us up no end, and shopped a little more. Ellie found a very style-y pair of leggings that look like jeans and a pink sweatshirt, which will be great in four months' time but are far too hot to wear now. Val bought a beautiful chiffon top perfect for wearing to Thalia's wedding – she resisted buying it at first, but Ellie and I told her firmly that even if she's dreading the whole thing it will be much better to be miserable while looking good. I bought a very nice pair of shorts and a polka-dotted shirt, entirely by accident; I wasn't meant to be shopping for me.

By that time exhaustion had claimed us and we headed home via the supermarket. We got home at five, completely shattered. I don't understand why a day in Hamilton is more tiring than a day pregnancy-testing, but it really is.

Sunday 2 February

We realised this morning that if we didn't vasectomise any rams now it would be too late (they're still fertile for up to a month after the surgery). It would have been better to do it in November, when things were cool and green and fresh rather than hot and dusty and swarming with flies, but since it was now or never, we decided it had better be now.

It went very well – which is always a relief, with surgery; there are so many ways it can go wrong. The patient won't go to sleep, or (hideous thought) the patient won't wake up, or you nick a blood vessel and obscure the surgical field, or you can't decide whether the squishy, bleeding bit of tissue in front of you is, in fact, the bit that you want, because it looks nothing like the picture in the textbook …

But today everything went like clockwork. The rams went quietly to sleep, James tipped them up and I cleaned their scrotums, injected them with local, made a small, neat incision over each testis and removed a section of sperm-delivery plumbing. Then we gave them a shot of antibiotic, sprayed them copiously to keep the flies off and sat them up again. I do love it when things go according to plan.

In the evening we went down to the river with two other families for a barbecue. The river is very low and very clear, and it's absolutely *teeming* with eels. I've never seen anything like it. If you waded into the water a couple would appear from nowhere and twine excitedly around your ankles. It was very cool to see, but somehow nobody felt very keen to swim.

We had a wonderful time. We ate and drank and paddled gingerly among the eels and skipped stones across the water, and when the sun had set we went for a walk along the flats and watched the moonlight shining on the river. The kids picked blackberries and toasted marshmallows and fed leftover sausages to the eels. There were glow worms all along the banks under the ladder fern as we drove up the track through the bush.

We are so, so lucky to live here.

Monday 3 February

First day back at school. The kids were both up and dressed with lunchboxes packed by quarter to seven. I do hope they're starting the way they mean to go on.

Unlike them I didn't go to work today – I'm vetting Wednesday to Friday this month instead of Monday to Wednesday, because we have a locum helping with scanning who can only work Mondays and Tuesdays, and it seemed more sensible to work on days that she can't. Logically, working the last three days of the week should be the same as working the first three days, but there's something delightfully holiday-ish about not going to work on Monday.

This morning, James's great-uncle, who is 98 and looks good for at least another ten years, brought down a juvenile wood pigeon his neighbour found sitting on the ground last night. This dry weather is awfully hard on young birds. It had spent the night in a cardboard box with a dish of water, and it came out bright-eyed and pissed off, which I thought was an excellent sign. I checked it over for broken bones (none), poked peas into its mouth until it stopped swallowing them (about 40), gave it a long drink of water from a syringe and a shot of antibiotic in case it had some internal infection, and Uncle John took it home again to release on familiar territory.

After he had gone, I went out to collect faecal samples from mobs of calves – a pleasant, if not glamorous, way to spend a morning. With any luck, you find the mob sitting somewhere in the shade, and approach quietly. When you get fairly close, they all get to their feet, stretch, poo and wander off. Then you scurry from one fresh cowpat to the next, collecting three teaspoonfuls from each and tipping them into a ziplock bag ready to send off to the lab.

I got home feeling industrious and generally pleased with myself, put my faecal samples in the fridge (double-wrapped) and, in a misplaced burst of enthusiasm, went back out into the burning sun to spray some more tradescantia. At 2 p.m. I crawled limply back home, hot, scratched, pink with spray dye from ankle to knee and generally having lost the will to live. James had just got in from feeding out and was in very much the same state. Summer is great if you're lounging by the sea, but highly overrated for working in.

Tuesday 4 February

Spend from 1.15 to 1.55 a.m. up with Blake, who woke up with an alleged sore throat and then threw up copiously. We sat on the bathroom floor, him conveniently close to the toilet bowl, while I read him *The Wee Free Men* to take his mind off his sufferings.

This morning he bounded out of bed, ate a large breakfast and insisted he'd never felt better and that his life would be blighted if he didn't go to school. I let him go, although my conscience is giving me some twinges. But surely it can't be anything catching – who ever heard of a 45-minute bug?

I just waylaid James on his way out the door to go to town and suggested he change his outfit. He'd swapped his farm clothes for a highlighter-yellow camo-patterned T-shirt and red-and-blue-striped swimming shorts, plucked at random from the clean washing pile. James is totally oblivious to fashion. His favourite hat, for example, is a horrible knitted cap with earflaps that makes him look like Tweedledum, which was given to him as a joke.

Wednesday 5 February

What a horrendous day. I spent most of it in a state of total panic, trying to do seventeen things at once and thus cocking most of them up.

I knew today would be a big day, so I thought I'd go to work early and get a head start. Accordingly, at seven thirty I kissed the family goodbye and got into the ute. The clock on the dashboard said 7.46, and my phone confirmed it; my watch was slow. At that point I found three recently missed calls from the after-hours lady, wanting me to go and look at a colicky horse. I'd turned my phone to silent by mistake. I called her back, and found that she'd already called someone else to go and look at it – Bill, who had the day off. Bugger.

At the clinic I flew from one job to the next, putting my surgery kit in to soak, filling out export declaration paperwork and emailing it, tossing vaccine into chilly bins, ringing people with last week's lab results. In this flurry of activity, I neglected to put a scanner into my ute. I was already running late when I went back to the clinic to get it, couldn't find it (although it was in the normal place) and spent another five minutes running around the building like a headless chicken, accusing my colleagues of collective theft and/or negligence. Just to complete the debacle, on the way out of town I scuttled into the post office with a parcel containing Monday's bag of calf poo, which absolutely *had* to catch the morning mail pick-up to get to the lab that day, and they told me they weren't the depot for that particular courier company. It took me most of the drive to my first job to stop twitching and hyperventilating.

I was actually only fashionably (five minutes) rather than unprofessionally (ten minutes) late, and the scanning job went very well – nice cool breeze, nice roomy cowshed, nice quiet cows. But then I arrived at my second job to find that I'd brought the wrong vaccine with me. I called the clinic and Jess rushed out with more.

I got back in around three, pausing to collect James's work boots from a shop where he'd left them yesterday. (He kicked them off at the door and drove home in his socks without noticing. Nice to know I'm not the only one in the family losing my mind.) There I spent half an hour I couldn't spare talking to a farmer at the front counter – supposedly because he wanted advice, but actually because he wanted to tell me how much better his farming operation is than James's and mine.

I saw a dog with a high fever and no other clinical signs – always worrying; perhaps the signs were there and I missed them. I asked Melissa to have a look at it, and she thought its lungs sounded wheezy. Filled it up with antibiotics, anti-inflammatories and subcutaneous fluids – tomorrow is a public holiday, so no point in taking bloods. Gave the owner my cell phone number in case it doesn't make a miraculous recovery overnight.

Rushed out to revisit two dearly beloved sick goats, which have neurological problems after eating mouldy scraps and were bedded down in the client's living room. Gave them antibiotics, fluids and pain relief. It was only on returning to the clinic that I learnt they took ill on Friday and have deteriorated since, despite treatment, and that I really should have put the poor things down.

I got back to work just on five, paperwork still incomplete, to find everyone else sitting limply around in reception. Nobody else had any lunch today either; everyone is feeling hot and bothered and overworked. Ah, pregnancy-testing season. If only it was in July rather than February, when you'd be *grateful* to dress in gumboots, waterproof overalls and long gloves, and plunge to the shoulder into a nice warm cow.

Thursday 6 February
Waitangi Day. Public holiday. Thank God.

This morning I delivered Ellie to her best friend's house, went to the supermarket for camping supplies and picked up Blake's friend on the way home. At the mailbox we met Dan, who told us that the helicopter working just down the hill has been commissioned by the police to spray somebody's marijuana plantation. Most exciting.

Excitement notwithstanding, Dan's looking tired and flat. Which is not surprising – he's been getting up before five every morning for the last seven months, his ex-girlfriend is now going out with the manager of the pub and telling anyone who'll listen that he's The One, and there's no rain forecast for the next fortnight. I asked him to come down the river after milking on Saturday and stay for a barbecue. He was noncommittal but I *think* he was pleased to be asked – it's hard to tell with Dan.

As soon as we got home the boys put on a motorbike helmet each and vanished down the orchard. Nice to see them so safety conscious, but I was slightly saddened when, at lunchtime, Blake's friend remarked that he's had nits for *months* and *nothing* seems to kill them. Sprayed the inside of Ellie's helmet liberally with fly spray and hoped for the best.

After lunch I delivered both boys to the epic waterslide built by Blake's friend's uncle. (Blake tells me that Uncle Josh is the best uncle *ever* – he showed Blake how to give mean wedgies and how to pinch someone on the soft skin just below their armpit for maximum pain. Neat.) I got back home just as James did, and we went out to spend some quality time together battening a fence. It was very nice too. After our fence battening we went to inspect the patch of jasmine I've been trying to kill, which is dying nicely in some spots but still flourishing in many others, and as we stood there wondering where next to attack it, a whole family of tomtits – mum, dad and two teenagers – came to see what we were doing. Tomtits are adorable.

Thalia and Adam came for dinner to discuss wedding planning. They're taking the whole week before their wedding off, and will come on Thursday with various friends to put up a marquee and erect and decorate a rustic archway at the end of the wide grass path, beneath the albizia tree. We're not to do a thing, not even mow the lawn. They're perfectly happy with the garden – or at least they're excellent actors – and say it's looking better than they could have dreamt, considering the last six weeks of burning sun. It doesn't matter, they insist, that the lawn looks like the African savannah; it just makes the trees look greener and fresher by contrast.

Friday 7 February

Up at four for an early morning scanning job in a rotary cow shed on the other side of town – 600 cows, with cups on at 5 a.m. I don't mind early jobs (much), but I'm so glad I don't work in the South Island, where most of the scanning jobs are early morning ones and the average herd size is over 1000 cows. I suspect the novelty would wear off quite quickly.

Back at the clinic, I had a long to-do list and was looking forward to cracking on with it when a call came in to see a cow who'd been stabbed for bloat on the wrong side. (Stabbing a cow on the left side is a life-saving procedure, resulting in a relatively easy-to-sew-up hole in the rumen; stabbing one on the right just leads to holes in goodness only knows what bit of intestine, most likely followed by peritonitis and death.) Everybody else pleaded extreme busyness and said they couldn't go until the afternoon, so I went, in a most unattractive mood of self-righteous martyrdom.

When I arrived, I found that the cow had been stabbed a week ago, and her abdominal organs were now set, like one of those nasty gelatine moulds people served at dinner parties back in the seventies, in a mass of fibrin. I asked the farm manager to go home for his gun and shoot her – he was most put out at the cow's ingratitude in dying of peritonitis when he'd spent six hours nursing her the week before. I'd have thought, personally, that the cow had more grounds for complaint about the situation than he did.

*

After work I collected the children from their friends' houses and spent a couple of hours packing feverishly to go camping, wondering, as always, if the camping could possibly be worth the effort. James got home at five thirty, Clare arrived at six, and we loaded most of the contents of the house onto the back of the ute and headed for the river, meeting another family at the top of the track.

An hour later the tents were set up, the children were bonding with the tame eels and the adults were reclining in the evening sunlight, chilled beverages in hand, the murmur of water filling our ears. *Totally* worth the effort.

Sunday 9 February, 9 p.m.

Sitting on the couch, sunburnt and exhausted, while the third load of washing spins in the machine.

It's been a great weekend. The logistics of getting organised to go camping are moderately horrible, but once you're there, there's no cell phone coverage and nothing to do except sleep and swim and pick blackberries if you're feeling energetic. (For breakfast this morning we had pancakes with blackberry compote – it was exceptionally classy.) Our friends' daughters have suddenly hit their teens and wished only to huddle giggling in their tent listening to music, but although they couldn't be bothered talking to the rest of us, they weren't actively hostile, so who cares? And we forgot the axe and had to cut the firewood with a drainage spade, but it was good exercise.

Dan actually did come down on Saturday night. He looked nervous when he arrived, and was obviously wishing he'd stayed home, but Blake attached himself to his side like a delighted limpet and covered the awkward introduction phase. Then Clare sat down beside him on a log and plied him with beer and attention, and he unfolded like a rosebud. (Not sure that's the metaphor I want; it sounds vaguely obscene.) After dinner we strolled along the riverbank looking for bats and admiring swooping wood pigeons and rising trout and the changing colours of the bush as the sun went down. Then we reclined in comfort around the fire for a while until the moon rose, when we walked up the bush track to see the glow worms, Clare and Dan well to the rear. It was a gorgeous night, warm and still, the glow worms glowed like a carnival and the silhouette of the pungas against the moon was breathtaking. I've never seen a night so drenched in romance – it practically oozed out of the air. Finally Dan left, looking dazed and bewildered, and Clare went for a solitary walk downriver to commune with the moon. I am trying hard not to marry them in my imagination, and settle my best friend 500 metres down the road. We could go walking in the evenings, and she could revitalise the small-animal department at work, and ... Stop it.

Monday 10 February

Flow-like writing state this morning interrupted by scraping sounds from laundry. Investigated and found Bean the cat trying, very tidily, to dig a hole in the floor and bury a small pile of regurgitated cat biscuits. Her mistaking the lino for a patch of dirt was entirely understandable. Removed vomit and spent ten minutes scrubbing the floor with concentrated bleach and a stiff brush. The house now smells like a men's public toilet, but the laundry floor looks *pristine*. And at least it smells like a *clean* men's public toilet. It could be infinitely worse.

Sunday 16 February

Just opened emails to find weekly pasture growth predictions. One kilogram of dry matter per hectare per day for the foreseeable future. (In November we grow 40.) This drought is getting kind of dire. The hills are turning from buff to silvery grey, without the faintest tinge of green.

I haven't written anything for almost a week. Monday and Tuesday we dipped and condition scored ewes; Wednesday to Friday I scanned cows. Four or five hundred a day, with cats and dogs and lame cows and a random oystercatcher with a broken beak in between. James is feeding out ten bales of silage a day – it's good silage and we're very grateful to have plenty on hand, but he gets very little else done. Thursday was Ellie's birthday and we went out for Indian; on Friday afternoon my aunt and uncle came to stay the night.

They're terribly health conscious, and talk at length about their abstinence from red meat, alcohol, sugar and caffeine, but they seem to be able to worry it all down at our place. They get around the inconsistency by accepting glasses of wine, cups of coffee and second helpings of roast potatoes with reluctant distaste. These conversations go like this:

'Would you like a hot drink, Uncle Bevan?'

'Hmm? Oh, alright.'

'What would you like?'

'Oh, er, I'll have a coffee, then. But just a small one.'

Or, as I pour myself a glass of wine:

'Wine, Aunty Brenda?'

(*Sighs*) 'Very well.'

It's not like I don't offer them anything healthy. I made sure to serve a large green salad with dinner – they took one small lettuce leaf apiece, and had seconds of roast mutton. Just saying.

Yesterday we had Ellie's birthday afternoon tea. She decided to have just family this year rather than friends – Val, Thomas, Diane and the girls, and Amy and her girls, who after living next door for five years count as family. The party was an uproarious success, largely thanks to the epic failure of the cake. Ellie asked for cheesecake, and I made an enormous one with a plum topping. I had more stewed plums than the recipe called for, and less gelatine, but I thought it would set alright in the fridge.

It didn't. When transferred from cake tin to serving platter the whole thing quivered, sagged, and then the topping flowed gently off the top of the cheesecake, across the dish and onto the table. It looked absolutely revolting. Like an enormous ruptured abscess. But everyone thought it was hilarious, and it tasted good, and the children very kindly sucked the escaping topping off the table with smoothie straws before it engulfed the ice-cream sandwiches.

Monday 17 February

An exhausting day. This morning I spent two hours helping James drench and dip lambs in the choking dust (such a catch 22 – yarding lambs in the dust is a leading cause of pneumonia, but leaving them to be eaten by worms and flies isn't ideal either). Then we had a cup of coffee and parted ways, him to feed out and me to spray tradescantia right at the back of the farm in a steep gully above a series of waterfalls. For anyone wanting to get fit, I can really recommend climbing up and down rock faces with a twenty-litre sprayer on your back. As I sprayed, I listened to *My Dad Wrote a Porno*, the only podcast that was already downloaded onto my phone. It's very funny, but is, I find, best taken in smaller amounts. After three episodes of the ghastly Belinda's improbable sexual antics I felt like the inside of my head needed a good scrub with soap and hot water, and turned it off. I sprayed on until I hooked the wand of the sprayer around a branch and broke it, and then took off all my clothes and lay face down in the creek. Which was absolutely lovely, until I remembered that the pool I was lying in was the one where James's uncle was once bitten by an enormous eel, taking a chunk of flesh right out of his calf.

I climbed out again, staggered up the hill to the ute and drove home, where I stripped at the door to put my clothes straight into the wash. The machine was full of clean washing, so I emptied it and hung it out. And as I stood naked at the washing line Thomas whirled up the driveway on his motorbike and caught me like a rabbit in the headlights. Reacting completely differently to the way that Belinda would have, I dashed around the corner of the house and in through the French doors just in time to hear him roar off again. Why did it have to be *Thomas*, of all people? He'll probably never be able to look me in the face again. Although, let's be honest, he barely looked me in the face anyway. It can't make much difference.

Ellie and I were in her bedroom after school, sorting clothes to go to the op shop, when Blake ran in, shouted, 'You shall not pass!', farted and ran out again. Ellie was understandably incensed by this behaviour, but as I pointed out, it could have been worse. He could have farted and stayed.

Amy just told me that tonic water contains as much sugar as lemonade. And there I thought that gin and tonic was delicious *and* low in calories. It's a crushing blow.

Tuesday 18 February

James is as cranky as a cranky thing. Not without justification – it's stinking hot, he's spending four hours a day on the tractor and they keep forecasting rain for five days' time and then changing their minds two days out – but it's a little wearing.

This morning we were dipping and vaccinating the ewe lambs when one turned around in the race, as they do, and he snarled, 'It's all very well that *you* wanted to save money, but *I'm* the one who has all the extra work. *I'm* the one who has to tow the bloody dipping race out here and spend three hours mustering. Maybe next year we'll just spend the money and do it once, properly.'

Now, I'm pretty sure I remember our conversation about whether to treat the sheep with the four-months-prevention chemical at two dollars apiece, or whether to run them through the dip every two months for 30 cents, and, if I recall, his comment *then* was, 'It's a lot cheaper to run them through the dip. And they have to come in for drenching anyway.'

But I just murmured something soothing, and we carried on. We had finished the job and were returning the lambs from whence they came when he ordered: 'Go in front of the lambs and open the gate for them out of the Near Dam.'

'Which gate?' (There are four.)

'Into the Big Face.'

'But there are two ... Sorry, where do you mean exactly?'

(Deep sigh.) 'Oh, don't worry, it's easier to do it all myself. As usual.'

'No, hang on. Tell me again.'

'The – gate – from – the – Near – Dam – into – the – Big – Face.' (Said through his teeth.) 'There's only one.'

'But I'm sure there are two!'

'Nope.'

'There's the one by the big poplars and the one down by the hay barn.' (The Big Face is divided into five paddocks, and those two gates open into different paddocks.)

'Well, not the one by the hay barn, *obviously*.'

Right. Obviously not.

Wednesday 19 February

Scanned 600 cows. Temperature 28 degrees, humidity 100 percent. Our goggles fogged up, we were drenched in sweat and the cow shed was a spectacularly awkward one, with cup removers and milk lines and random pipework in the way wherever we turned. It felt like one of those hardcore hot yoga classes. Whew.

Thursday 20 February

Got up at five thirty, paid bills, reconciled accounts, filed a GST return. Drove for an hour to a distant and very beautiful corner of the district to scan 400 heifers. A nice job – the farm manager is a lovely chap, and he'd organised extra help in the shape of a delightful couple who live next door. They both wore full cowboy regalia – button-down checked shirts, jeans, ten-gallon hats, shiny belts and cowboy boots. Now *that* is impressive dedication to style. They must have *cooked* in those outfits. They looked great, though.

Continued to neighbouring farm, eating a marmite sandwich and two plums on the way, and scanned another 600 heifers – this time with Ben, the clinic manager, helping, since the race was long enough for two vets. He very kindly took the front of the race, which has higher sides and is more awkward than the back. Finished at four, cleaned up and drove an hour home, stopping on the way to see a lame calf.

I was so tired I couldn't get to sleep when I went to bed. Got up and wandered distractedly around the house, making plaintive, incoherent grizzling sounds when James spoke to me.

Friday 21 February

Slight hiccup at the office this morning when Melissa reached her first scanning job, assembled her scanner and found there were no goggles in the box. She rushed back into the clinic, where we hunted high and low until I had a thought and called yesterday's heifer job.

'Yep,' the farmer said. 'They're here, sitting on the post where you left them.'

Oh dear oh dear oh dear.

Sunday 23 February

Spent the weekend gardening – trimming edges, dead-heading and pulling out summer grass, which somehow manages to keep growing without water. There are, miraculously, some pretty spots – the orchard is still greenish, and there's a nice patch of red tussock and sedums and gloriosa lilies that actually looks quite stylish.

Ellie is nursing another wood pigeon – James found it sitting on the ground down by the creek yesterday, exhausted and starving, and brought it home wrapped in his shirt. It's now living in Ellie's bedroom, in the inner shell of a two-man tent beside her bed, and is already tame enough to take peas from her hand.

I just spent half an hour wiping all the skirting boards in the house, after an acquaintance told me that the tenants have just moved out of her rental property. 'I refused to refund their bond,' she said. 'Would you believe they never cleaned the skirting boards *once*?'

A moment's reflection confirmed that I'd never cleaned a skirting board in my life – the eye-level dirt takes up more than enough of my time. Our skirting boards were indeed pretty grubby. They are now, however, immaculate.

Monday 24 February

The pigeon was dead this morning. Ellie is broken-hearted. Did I miss some treatable condition, or was the poor thing just too far gone? It was a bit flat last night, but I thought it probably just had a sore stomach from the unaccustomed food. Damn it.

*

I spent all morning in the bush filling bait stations with the very nice neighbour who has helped us with them for years but has now decided it's time to hand the job on and is teaching me where his bait lines run. Since he's 80 and has chronic asthma, this is inarguably fair enough. Between eight and one we climbed up ridges and slithered down banks, by which time I was exhausted. Also quite humbled, when I reflected that he's twice my age and has half my lung capacity.

It's horribly dry in the bush. The begonia fern, normally so dense and lush, is like piles of limp rubber hose across the ground, and all the little seedlings are drooping unhappily. Apart from two fantails, and three wetas in an empty bait station, we saw not a single bird or insect.

James wasn't home when I got back for lunch, and as I ate a solitary bowl of Weet-Bix I reflected on all the things wrong with the world. This horrible drought will become a near-annual experience, thanks to global warming. And honestly, what is the point of messing around trying to poison a few possums and spray a few weeds when there are billions too many people in the world, and large bits of Australia are on fire, and they're *still* cutting down the Amazon rainforest just as fast as they can? Not to mention that Thalia's wedding is on Saturday and I don't like my haircut, and my hands are all scratched, with skin like a lizard's …

At that point, luckily, my blood sugar levels started to rise, and James got home, and I decided that things may not, after all, be entirely and irrevocably hopeless.

Tuesday 25 February

Blake, who is reading my computer screen from beside me on the couch, says that Blake is a dumb name for a boy in a book and I should change it.

'To what?' I ask.

'Captain Cook.'

'Er, no.'

'What about Legolas of the Woodland Realm?'

Clare texted last night to ask if she could come and stay this weekend. I had to put her off because of the wedding. Suggested that Dan would probably be delighted to put her up, and received a middle-finger emoji in return.

Wednesday 26 February

Ridiculously hot day. The morning's scanning job was fine, but then I spent from twelve thirty to two scanning heifers in a crumbling race beneath the burning sun, overseen by an apathetic, grizzling dairy farmer, and I nearly lost the will to live.

I went home for a cool shower and a cold drink, and then picked the kids up from school to go back into town for Ellie's dance class. While she danced, Blake and I bought three ice creams and took one to James's great-aunt, who has recently moved from her own house into care. Transporting ice-cream cones in the summer heat is a risky undertaking, but the dairy is close to the home and I was feeling confident.

We managed, but it was a close call. The ice cream was a bit soft already, and the dairy owner asked me a lot of searching questions about whether his dog might have an ear infection while I was trying to pay. Eventually we escaped and flew along the main street, ice cream dripping from our wrists (we weren't sure what flavour, if any, Aunty Sue would want, so we didn't like to start licking any of them). We burst through the doors of the home, galloped across the lounge to Aunty Sue's chair and brandished a row of wilting ice creams at her. She rose to the occasion nobly, seized the mint chocolate chip cone and applied herself to it without wasting a second. Conversation was out of the question for a few minutes, but once we'd dealt with the ice cream and mopped ourselves up a bit, we had a lovely visit. Blake insisted on spreading out his collection of Pokémon cards and explaining each one's powers, and he and Aunty Sue discussed them with absorbed interest. She really *was* interested, too. If I try really hard, I wonder if I could get as nice as her by the age of 89?

Thursday 27 February

Wonderful news! The awful, stiff, mutually hurt-feelinged chill between Val and Thalia is thawing. Not before time. Last night, apparently, Val found Thalia in tears and hugged her, and Thalia wept all over her and apologised for being so difficult and said that Trevor seems very nice. Oh, thank God.

On the way to work this morning I passed Dan in his tractor. He looked the picture of gloom. Right, I thought, and pulled off the road to text him Clare's number, with the message: *I'm pretty sure she likes you.* Of course, I bitterly regretted interfering the second I'd sent it, but it was too late.

He hasn't replied. Probably not surprising.

Friday 28 February

Adam and the two groomsmen are staying at our house tonight. They're charmingly polite and helpful, with identical haircuts, and the kids are beside themselves with excitement at the privilege of sleeping on the lawn in a tent while these gods occupy their bedrooms. Slightly less charming is Adam's brother's girlfriend, who wasn't actually supposed to be staying until tomorrow night but decided that whither Adam's brother goest, she's damn well going too. Her stay got off to a slightly rocky start when the back doorhandle came off in her hand. I assured her it's been like that for months – we forget, because we've learnt the trick of opening it – and her eyebrows rose slightly. They rose a lot further when she wanted a shower and the bathroom lights wouldn't come on. The last bulb blew a week ago, and they're unusual bulbs that aren't available any closer than Hamilton, and frankly it hasn't been a priority. I've actually quite enjoyed not being able to see my face in the mornings as I brush my hair and put on my moisturiser. I explained this, and she looked me up and down as if she could completely see my point.

Autumn

Autumn is gorgeous. Hands down my favourite season. It contains mushroom rings and autumn crocuses and spider webs starred with dew and mellow golden sunsets and cool, misty mornings ...

Unless there's a drought, in which case it doesn't.

Sunday 1 March

The house is temporarily empty, except for me – James is feeding out, and the bridal party have taken the kids up to Val's for lunch and the post-wedding debrief. James and I will go up too, when he gets home – in the meantime I could start stripping beds and cleaning the toilet (which, sadly, many, many people used last night instead of the portaloos). But I'm going to sit here drinking coffee instead and worry about it later. So there.

The wedding went off beautifully. Lovely ceremony, lovely food, champagne and laughter and overflowing goodwill on every side. Thalia looked gorgeous, and the hairdresser who'd come to do the bridal party's hair very kindly spent ten minutes blow-drying mine. Blake ran past as she finished, stopped dead and said, 'Wow, Mum! You look beautiful!' Which was heartening, although it's a shame that he followed it up with, 'You look so much better than normal!'

Val gave a *superb* mother-of-the-bride speech. It was funny, and touching – and brief, which is *very* important. In it she explained that she'd been guided by the words of Winston Churchill: 'A good speech should be like a woman's skirt; long enough to cover the subject and short enough to create interest.'

Adam's speech was very funny too – in the stress of the moment, he forgot Thalia's name and said, 'And my lovely wife … um, my lovely wife … shit, I have a wife …'

James and Ellie danced for two hours straight – they both, unlike Blake and me, have rhythm and style. They were awesome. Also slightly dangerous to passers-by. I will always treasure the image of them flossing in perfect synchrony.

And I had a brief and absolutely staggering conversation with Thomas.

We were temporarily the only ones at the table, and I was just going to get up and mingle so as not to sit there in uncomfortable silence when he leant towards me and whispered, 'I'm a li'l bit drunk. Don' tell Diane.'

'No, I won't,' I said.

'I know. You're always kind.'

Mildly shocked, I smiled modestly and started pushing back my chair.

And *then* he said, 'You know what? I was gon' ask you out when you firs' came and calved that cow for Dad. But then James did.'

I sat and looked at him with my mouth open for a while, and then croaked, 'But you don't like me!'

'Huh?'

'You don't even talk to me!'

''S safer not to,' he said solemnly, and got up and wandered away, weaving slightly.

Good Lord. I'm shocked and stunned. And a little bit pleased, and a little bit sad, and … Best not to think about it. Although of course I will.

Monday 2 March

Work today – I'm back to working the start rather than the end of the week. As we were cleaning up from this morning's scanning job, I heard the farmer giving instructions to his worker on where to put the cows.

'Oh, just go for a drive up the race,' he said, 'and pick a paddock that you think has a nice view.' (He's feeding out, of course – the poor cows aren't making do with just the insignificant few bits of dead stalk left in the paddocks.)

If only it would rain! Once more the forecast for heavy rain at the end of the week has been downgraded to 'a few showers' on Wednesday morning. And I'll believe those when I see them.

But to think of happier things, there was a tomtit in the garden this morning! Ellie has taken multiple photos of it, bouncing around in the little magnolia in front of the kitchen window. I think it's a baby – it has a very short tail. Tomtits are the sweetest little birds ever: black and white, with big heads and little stubby bodies; very friendly, very curious. Bean hasn't caught a bird for years, but I'm withholding her arthritis medication to make absolutely sure. Callous, I know, but there it is. (I salve my conscience with the thought that at least I'm not as mean as the lady who told me last week that her old cat shat in her wardrobe, so she kicked it out and now it lives in the bush. I did like her, but now I'm not so sure.)

Tuesday 3 March

We just watched a Michael Moore documentary about various things that are wrong with America. One of the areas he covered was the prison system. He went to Finland to look at their prisons; safe, pleasant places where the inmates are taught to become useful members of society when they come out. And then the segment closed with footage taken in American prisons. There was clip after clip of guards savagely beating inmates; throwing them unconscious into concrete cells; setting dogs on them. Most of those prisoners looked really, really young. It made me cry. How the hell is that supposed to teach them anything except hate?

Ellie and I are reading *Carpe Jugulum* at bedtimes, and tonight we got to the bit where Granny Weatherwax says that all sin starts with treating people as things. As usual, Terry Pratchett absolutely nailed it.

Wednesday 4 March

It's our wedding anniversary today! We've been married for fourteen whole years. We didn't feel like going out to celebrate – we're still recovering from the weekend – but we had potato cakes and bacon for tea, and agreed that getting married was a good decision and if we could go back in time, we'd do it again.

James is very pleased with himself this evening – he's just finished a niggly little bit of fence. He laid the posts out twelve years ago, rammed them in a couple of years later, moved them a couple of years after that, and finally put the wires up this afternoon. Good things take time.

I had a good day too. I was on small-animal surgery rather than cow pregnancy-testing, and today's patients were especially nice.

There was a young farm dog for castration, so eager to please that he wet himself whenever we patted him, and an elderly Bichon Frisé with terrible teeth who just wanted to snuggle. Sophie and I drained at least half a litre of pus from the cheek of another charming farm dog (I adore lancing abscesses; so satisfying), and to top it all off, a truck driver brought in his pet sparrow, worried it had lost its chirp. How cute is that?

Thursday 5 March

Amy and the girls came for afternoon tea after school for the first time in ages. Amy was a bit limp today – a combination of her period being due tomorrow and her children waking through the night. She brought three hand-me-down tops for Ellie, and I gave her a wetsuit Blake has grown out of and half the mince I'd made for tea, since she wasn't feeling strong enough to cook. The warm glow of doing something nice for a friend more than compensates for the loss of tomorrow night's potential shepherd's pie.

Friday 6 March

I went out early to fill a few bait stations, and got back very concerned about the lambs I'd encountered on my travels. There's no green grass at all now; the poor things are making do with dried stem. I told James they'd have to be moved and so he drove that way to do it. He rang me half an hour after leaving home to say bitterly that he *had* moved them, but they'd actually been in the best grass on the farm.

No rain is forecast for the next two weeks.

*

I went into town and had a facial today, which seems appallingly frivolous in the face of disastrous drought. It was lovely, though, lying back in comfort while Nicolette smoothed cool creams onto my face and muttered under her breath at my obstreperous left eyebrow, which has a kink in it and will *not* be made into a graceful arch.

I floated out to the car after my facial, and found three increasingly distressed messages on my phone – a very valuable breeding kiwi that is currently incubating an egg was caught on camera last night choking, vomiting and staggering around in his enclosure. He obviously needed to go to the wildlife hospital at Massey, but should be triaged first and given fluids and pain relief before the trip. I'd planned to go to school assembly, at Blake's request, but this obviously wasn't something that could be put off. I flew into work and feverishly read the *Kiwi Husbandry Manual* while waiting for the patient to arrive.

He duly turned up, and we discovered that the inside of his mouth was caked with dried food. The new captive kiwi diet is quite sticky, and people all over the country are having problems with it. I picked the plaques of food out with a fingernail while he glared at me and rattled his beak. We agreed that the apparent choking was probably an attempt to clear his mouth, and the keepers hurried him back to his egg. Crisis de-escalated. Whew.

And since the kiwi crisis only took ten minutes, I still made it to assembly. Which was good, since Ellie was MC-ing it and Blake was presenting interesting facts about sharks. As usual, assembly was almost unbearably cute. Today's song was 'Roar' by

Katy Perry, which the girls (including me) sang enthusiastically and the boys endured, and then the principal gave a very nice, very gentle little talk about how if you decide you'd like to play ball tag at lunchtime, it's a little bit unreasonable to then rush up to the teachers and tell on the person who just hit you with a ball.

We'd only just got home when our awesome neighbour Shane, who gave us the calves, rang from the paddock below the house to see where we'd like him to put the new swimming pool. This sounds much more glamorous than it really is – the pool is a big square cattle trough, 2 metres wide, 4 metres long and about 70 centimetres deep. I had a brainwave a few weeks ago, inspired by an episode of *Gardener's World* and a week of daytime temperatures over 30 degrees, and thought that if we put a concrete trough just downstream from the little spring below the woolshed, under the culvert pipe that runs beneath the crossing, we'd have a lovely, self-cleaning pool at the head of the swamp. (Having had the initial idea, I've done nothing more about the project; James and Shane have masterminded the whole thing.)

The kids and I went down and watched while Shane scraped a flat place with his digger bucket and dropped the trough into it. He even recontoured the bank while he was at it. A dozen freshwater crayfish were uncovered in the process, and Ellie carefully carried them to safety.

It's fantastic! Of course, it's not a real swimming pool, but it will do a very nice job of cooling us off in hot weather. The water pours in at one end and gently overflows on the far side. And when I plant ferns and trees all around it, it will be beautiful.

9 p.m.

I've just been emailed a contract which details the conduct expected from me at a book festival I've been invited to in June. It's pages long, and informs me (among many other stipulations) that I must refrain from defacing public property and from offensive behaviour that may bring the organisers into disrepute. I'm not allowed to turn up drunk, use weapons, let off fireworks or say nasty things about them – or, in fact, say anything about them at all – on social media without their approval.

I don't mind signing it, I suppose – after all, I'm unlikely to be seized by the urge to write on their walls or masturbate on stage – but what an offensive document. No reasonable person would assume it was okay to act like that, and no *un*reasonable person would let signing the contract prevent them from being an arsehole if they felt like it. So, it's not just offensive to 99.9 percent of people; it's a waste of everyone's time. I hate pointless bureaucracy. Imagine if the person employed to write it had spent that time actually solving some problem, or even drawing a nice picture to go on the lunchroom fridge. That would have been much more useful.

When I become dictator of New Zealand, I shall implement a small test, to be taken in all workplaces before embarking on any new task. A very simple test, with a single question: *Will doing this make anything better?* Just think how much more people will accomplish, and how much better the accomplishments will be.

Sunday 8 March

We have given a couple of hundred heifers zinc boluses today, to stop them from getting facial eczema. It's a lousy job – the heifers don't, understandably, *like* having a great big applicator gun shoved down their throats, and they writhe and struggle and bash your hands against the sides of the race and hide their heads between their neighbours' legs so you can't reach them.

James had to feed out before we started; he said it'd be about eleven before he wanted me, then he called at ten to tell me to come straight out to the middle yards. I couldn't – I had a cake in the oven. A bad beginning.

The kids and I got there at ten thirty, and James swore at the heifers and at me until I told him he was acting like a dick and unloaded all the zinc boluses from the back of the ute ready to leave him to it and go home. Ellie and Blake helped me, half shocked that I was deserting Dad and half hopeful that they might not have to spend all day in the yards. James said nothing, but when I repented and started helping him with the next row, he went all quiet and sheepish and polite.

We got a good system going after our rocky start. Ellie chased the heifers up the race, Blake loaded the applicator guns and James and I bolused the heifers. We stopped for a picnic lunch between mobs – a very superior picnic lunch of peaches and plums and homemade wraps and an ice-cold beer – and finished at two. Then we went for a swim in the new pool on the way home. It actually ended up, against all expectation, being a fun day out for the whole family.

Monday 9 March

Rain today! Actual rain! James sent me the following series of text messages:

2.15 p.m. *13 mm!*
3.21 p.m. *How good is this rain*
3.43 p.m. *I cleaned out the spouting we will have a full tank of water in another 10 minutes*
4.10 p.m. *27 mm*
4.22 p.m. *33 mm!!!*

The rain was widespread – everyone got it – and everyone is giddy with delight.

There was a box of chocolates on my desk this morning, brought in by the man whose sparrow's chirp had gone squeaky.

For dinner tonight, James the Carbohydrate King made macaroni and diced boiled potato with grated cheese stirred through it and garlic bread.

An excellent day all round.

Wednesday 11 March

I pregnancy-tested Thomas and Diane's cows this morning. I don't usually do it; Bill is their preferred vet, but he's gone to Australia for a fortnight. Diane had a list of cows that had been synchronised and put up for AB in October, and she wanted to know if they had held to that insemination or been mated later by the bull.

'I can't tell you now, I'm afraid,' I said. 'That was five months ago, and we can only date them accurately for about the first three months of pregnancy. After that they just look enormous.'

'Oh,' she said. '*Bill* always dates them.'

I'm quite sure he doesn't, not in March. I explained that it's impossible to tell the difference between a 150-day pregnancy and a 120-day one – there's too much variation in foetal size – but I could tell she didn't believe me.

Thomas stayed at the back of the yards all the time I was there. I'm not sure if he remembers our chat at the wedding or was just following standard procedure in my presence. Anyway, I'm glad.

While running across the house paddock this evening, Blake stood on the mother of all thistles. He limped in, and Ellie and I spent a happy half-hour digging out as many as we could find. Almost nothing is as satisfying as digging out thistles – one tiny hole in the very top layer of skin, one squeeze, and out they spring.

I rang Clare tonight, and we had one of those unsatisfactory conversations where you're pretty sure the other person is checking their emails while talking to you. But she's coming down this weekend, so we'll catch up then.

Thursday 12 March

I've spent all the time the kids were at school being domestic while listening to an audiobook. A gripping book – Marian Keyes's latest. Accompanied by her soft Irish lilt I have:

- Delivered the kids' bikes to school ready for the annual triathlon tomorrow
- Made lasagne
- Stewed five kilos of apples

- Done two loads of washing
- Pruned the lemon tree
- Slashed back about an acre of tired-looking perennial phlox
- Picked up the piles of weeds and branches on the lawn (on the same day I put them there – unheard of)
- Helped James draft ewes before the rams go out on Sunday
- Resprayed the jasmine at the edge of the bush
- Taken the portable pump down to the quarry to refill a tank of water for a mob of heifers

The day flew by, but I have a strange, dazed, sleepwalking sort of feeling. I was there in body but not in spirit. I remind myself of a small child I met years ago. His mother claimed proudly that he ate up everything she offered him – and she was quite right, but the only way she could get him to eat at all was by putting *Mickey Mouse* on her iPad and spooning the food into him while his eyes were glued to the screen. I've never seen anything like it. Honestly, you could have fed that child mashed slugs, and I'm sure he'd never have noticed.

Dan's going to come for dinner on Saturday night, when Clare's here.

Friday 13 March, 6.45 a.m.
I've just spent half an hour lurching from fear, to panic, to flat-out despair, to wild relief. A most invigorating start to the morning.

I got up as usual at six, made myself a coffee, sat down on the couch with the laptop and opened the Word document of my manuscript. And up popped a horrible little dialogue box that read: *The selected file does not exist at this location. It may have been deleted, moved or renamed.*

I couldn't find it in recent documents – that is, I *could* find it, but it wouldn't open – or in recently deleted documents, or anywhere in my computer files. Google's instructions on how to restore lost documents drew a blank. My most recent copy was the one I sent to the publisher in November, about 30,000 words ago. Finally, in the calm of despair, I pressed some button or other and found it again. I don't know where it was, or what I did, or how to do it again if I have to – but never mind. I have now emailed myself a copy and saved one onto a memory stick.

I will back up regularly. I *will*.

8.30 p.m.

Marian Keyes and I spent a happy morning picking up silage wrap, loading it onto the back of the ute and piling it up in the middle hay barn. A surprisingly nice, clean job – James rolls up the wrap and stacks it tidily as he goes – although I met many quite large spiders.

I kept an eye on my watch so as to be early for the kids' triathlon, which started at eleven thirty. I was home at ten to eleven, got changed, made myself a cup of coffee – and then glanced at the wall clock and found it said 11.23 a.m. Which was surprising, because my wristwatch still said ten to eleven.

I flew down to school just in time for Blake's race (a distinct improvement on last year, when I missed it). He was well in the lead after the run, but started the bike ride in the wrong gear and slipped to the back of the pack. He finished fourth. He was sobbing and telling me he'd been sabotaged and it was everyone else's fault when the nice little boy who won came up to shake his hand. He refused. I gave him a Look. It must have been a properly scary Look, because he scuttled straight off to apologise.

At bedtime tonight we had a long talk about being a good sport, and how people who don't take responsibility for their own stuff-ups lead cramped, resentful, unhappy lives.

Saturday 14 March

I'm tired and feeling sorry for myself. I just tried to think of three nice things that happened today, and couldn't. So instead of counting my blessings, I'm going to slump and list my complaints.

- It was stinking hot today – last week's lovely rain already feels long ago and far away.
- My throat hurts. I expect I'm getting coronavirus.
- We're going to look into boarding school for Ellie, although we hate the idea. But the local high school sort of imploded last year, and it just doesn't sound like it's improving, even though the Ministry of Education stepped in and appointed someone official to sort it out. The year nine intake this year is down 50 percent. A neighbour whose daughter started there this year tells me that the kids can't understand a word that the teacher who takes them

for science and maths says because her English is so poor. A friend who was teaching there just left, saying she couldn't take it anymore. We don't want to send Ellie away – but on the other hand we'd quite like her to learn something.

- My bottom is covered in fine scratches, due to sliding down a very steep hill covered in long dead grass this morning, and failing to see the seedling gorse in time. Goodness only knows how the doctors will think I got them when I collapse with coronavirus and am rushed to hospital.
- Clare arrived at lunchtime, which should have been lovely but wasn't. She didn't feel like talking – at least, not to me. However, she and Ellie had a lovely time watching YouTube videos of someone squeezing maggots from a puppy's skin. As you do.
- James texted asking me to meet him at the middle yards at one with some lunch. I was running perfectly to schedule until he amended the time to one thirty. The extra half-hour undid me completely – I decided it would easily give me enough time to make the naan dough to go with tonight's curry, have a coffee, hang out the washing and clean the cutlery drawer. (Being slightly late is, I find, a great highlighter of household grime. I never notice the spots on the kitchen window unless I need to leave in 30 seconds, and then, all of a sudden, I can't put up with them a moment

longer.) And then Clare said she'd like to come too; she'd just get changed …

- We got to the middle yards at one forty, and found James, who'd been ready since one twenty, pacing in fury. We drafted ewes in an atmosphere of dust and strain, and then cut out a heifer who'd jumped the fence into a different mob. The heifers thoroughly enjoyed that. They kicked up their heels and chased the dogs, and allowed themselves to be mustered nearly to the gate before galloping past the motorbike back to the bottom of the hill. James was not a happy man. Clare, the kids and I headed thankfully for home, stopping en route to shovel half a tonne of palm kernel meal onto the ute and then back off into a bin to feed a mob of cattle. There is nothing nice about palm kernel. By buying it you're supporting the palm oil industry, which no decent person should want to do, and it's insanely dusty, so that you end up coated in a fine, choking layer of the stuff that sifts down out of your eyelashes into your eyes for hours afterwards. But we have no grass and limited silage, and the stock have to eat something.

I have digressed from specific grizzles to general whingeing. Back to bullet points:

- James didn't come home for dinner – too much feeding out to do.

- Dan *did* come for dinner. He was utterly lacking in cheerfulness or sparkle. The curry was a bit watery and a bit tough, due to being cooked fast and hot rather than long and slow. Clare was almost entirely silent. By the time Dan left at eight thirty I was shattered.
- And then the crowning insult: at eight forty-five Clare's phone buzzed, she read the message and said, 'Um, I'm just going to pop down to Dan's. See you later.' It turns out he came to visit her in Auckland the weekend of the wedding, and they got on like a house on fire, but being under my beady eye tonight depressed them both so much that they were totally bereft of speech. I wish they'd just *said*. If they'd vanished before dinner the kids and I could have had toasted sandwiches and watched *Shrek*, and everyone would have had a much nicer time.

Okay. Come on. Pulling myself together. Three nice things. Go.

- I never got polio and spent ten weeks in an iron lung and three years learning to walk again with crutches. (I've been reading *Over My Dead Body* by June Opie. What a classy human being she was.)
- Bean still loves me. She has assumed her normal position while I'm writing and is on my lap, tucked under my right elbow and purring.
- I can hear the motorbike. James is home.

Sunday 15 March

Clare returned at eleven forty-five this morning. She stayed for twenty minutes before leaving for lunch and a drive to the beach with Dan. I'm trying not to feel hurt, and failing.

Blake just wandered into the bathroom as I got out of the shower. 'What's that weird smell?' he asked.

'No idea,' I said.

A pause. 'Oh. Soap,' he said, and wandered off again.

I think I'd better start observing his washing routine in closer detail.

Thursday 19 March

It's been a strange and surreal week. The whole world is in a panic about coronavirus. As a nation we don't seem to have reached quite the levels of toilet-paper-hoarding madness as the Australians, but on Monday I did follow a couple around the supermarket who were pushing three trolleys between them. Maybe they have fourteen children and they always buy five boxes of Weet-Bix at a time. Maybe I did them an injustice by labelling them as selfish dickheads. Or maybe not.

Senior management at work sent a rather ill-thought-out guide to staff members on Tuesday. If there is any concern that a client is infected, the vets are to keep away while a nurse collects the animal and brings it into the consult room for examination. Nurses, we infer, are expendable.

Every organisation in the country, from the Vet Association to the bank to Sky TV, is sending out earnest emails detailing their plans for dealing with COVID-19. The National Fieldays, all conferences and sporting events have been suspended. So, to Blake's intense disgust, has the junior rugby muster, which he'd been looking forward to for weeks. To me that seems a real silver lining – a whole winter free from team sports! All those Saturday mornings *not* spent traversing the country to stand at the edges of various muddy fields! No sausage sizzles or cupcake stalls! Whoopee!

I am being too flippant. This is a big deal. People will die – and in some parts of the world they'll die unnecessarily, due to the medical system being overwhelmed. The financial repercussions will be awful. Just down the road the Kiwi House, which relies heavily on tour buses, is looking like closing for six months, with just a skeleton staff retained to feed the birds. It's frightening.

We have bitten the bullet and filled out an online enrolment form for Ellie to go to boarding school next year. They replied, requesting a personal, handwritten profile from Ellie about herself and why she wants to go. In her profile she wrote that her favourite things in all the world are dancing, taking photos and playing with eels. Will they be charmed by her originality, I wonder?

Friday 20 March

We have a possum in the lemon tree, judging by the half-dozen peeled lemons I found on the lawn this morning. Most insulting, considering the amount of time and effort I spend setting traps and filling bait stations. This afternoon Blake and I went up to Val's to borrow her excellent two-ended cage trap, and as we headed home, he said thoughtfully, 'I'd like to live in Nana's house when I grow up. I'll vacuum and weed the garden and everything.'

When I asked where Nana would live, he explained that she'd be so old by then that she'd be living in a home. I get the feeling that if it's up to Blake, poor Nana will be bundled off whether she wants to go or not.

I have learnt to use the front-end loader! James taught me how, so I can feed out the palm kernel on the days I'm not at work. I feel all smug and capable, like a McLeod's daughter. Maybe I should start wearing very tight jeans and a ten-gallon hat, so as to really look the part.

There's a stag roaring out the back of the farm – we can hear him from the washing line early in the morning. It's very inconvenient, because I really need to kick the tradescantia while it's down by spraying it again, but I am too much of a wimp to risk being skewered by a testosterone-crazed stag while I'm splashing up and down the creek.

Good joke James heard on the radio today:

> Q: What is red and sits in the corner?
> (I thought it was going to be one of those awful baby-with-a-potato-peeler jokes, but no …)
> A: A naughty strawberry.

Saturday 21 March

The possum in the lemon tree is dead. I couldn't figure out how to set the amazing double-ended cage trap, but last night

I heard the possum hissing and chattering his teeth, so I woke poor James from a sound sleep and sent him out to shoot it. A proper McLeod's daughter would no doubt have shot it herself, but never mind.

James and the kids went into town this morning and returned with a wide selection of presents (it's my birthday on Monday). They are:

- A large Castello Danish blue cheese
- A bottle of wine
- A packet of chocolate-covered gingernuts
- A tub of gourmet ice cream
- A state-of-the-art watering can
- A box of compost-heap starter
- A seed bell for birds

I have the nicest family in the world.

Monday 23 March

So, for my birthday this year, the prime minister has announced at least four weeks of total, nationwide, level-four lockdown, effective from midnight on Wednesday. All schools, restaurants and non-essential businesses will be closed. Everybody is to stay home if at all possible, in their own separate household bubbles, and there's to be no deciding to spend lockdown at the beach, tramping or hunting, no matter how socially distanced you plan to be. Emergency services will be quite busy enough without rescuing people from the consequences of their outdoor adventures, thank you very much.

Crikey.

I think it's a good precaution, though – much better than waiting for uncontrolled spread of infection and then getting really serious when it's too late. Poor, poor Italy, which is an awful warning of the worst-case scenario to the whole world.

The clinic is staying open – veterinary services are essential – but we're to work from home if humanly possible, and to visit farmers rather than them visiting us. I trialled this today, sitting down to call a list of farmers about their milk quality consults and to set up a remote login to the clinic server on my laptop, while Blake, who was home from school with a cold, hovered around me asking really urgent questions like, 'Mum, can you cut me some cheese?' and, 'Mum, can you come and watch how high I can kick my ball?' I have now established a temporary office in the spare room, with an If-the-door-is-shut-you-may-only-interrupt-if-you're-actually-on-fire policy.

In the afternoon we went out and shovelled palm kernel in the drizzle. Blake told me repeatedly how much fun he wasn't having until I roared, 'Yeah, well, it's my *birthday*, you selfish little prat!' and reduced him to sobbing remorse. Oops.

Mum appears to be spending all her time trawling Facebook for the latest information and forwarding it to me. I wish she wouldn't – I'm spending far too much time mindlessly reading news websites as it is. At five o'clock this evening I realised I'd just spent an hour pretending I was working but actually just skim-reading emails and getting increasingly panicky, and forced myself outside to plant the two beautiful rugosa roses Val gave me for my birthday. Thank goodness for gardening; it makes everything better.

We're starting homeschooling tomorrow. Blake and Ellie are both very excited about it, and we have written a schedule, selected special projects and printed off some maths worksheets. They've both set up desks in corners of their bedrooms, Blake's fenced off with pillows and reachable only by taking a flying leap off his bed. I confidently expect their enthusiasm to last for about seven minutes from the time that we start.

James made tea while I lay in the bath reading and drinking wine. Best husband ever.

Also, it rained on and off all day. I didn't pay this miracle the attention it deserved at the time, but it's FABULOUS.

Tuesday 24 March

The kids, as their writing assignment for day one of homeschooling, wrote to Aunty Sue, since we can't visit her. They gave me the letters to deliver when I go to town – Ellie has written *Don't worry I didn't lick the envelope* across hers.

Maths – Ellie long division, Blake multiplication. He had one wrong answer, so I marked him 29/30, precipitating an indignant lecture on the unfairness of not giving people a second chance when they make one tiny piddling mistake. Ellie's times tables are very shaky – a better parent would have known that already, I'm sure – so we made flash cards. She's now got her sixes and sevens nailed, and we're doing eights tomorrow.

Blake suggested he practise handwriting, rejected with scorn my suggestion that he copy a paragraph from our current bedtime book and wrote *pineaPle* fifty times. When I pointed out that pineapple has three p's and all of them sit neatly on their bottoms, he retreated to his room in a huff.

I told them to read for an hour and started my milk quality consults.

Farmer One hadn't filled in any of the required information and doesn't milk the cows himself so couldn't even take a guess at how many cases of mastitis they've had and what they treated them with. He promised to send me everything later, but as he always promises to get back to me and he never has yet, I'm not holding my breath.

Farmer Two cancelled on the grounds that there are more important things to worry about just now.

Farmer Three had scanned and emailed me all the information in advance. We had a pleasant and productive hour's chat about mastitis and animal health. Well, one out of three ain't bad.

After lunch I went into town to see a kiwi chick that's been regurgitating when hand-fed. The chick was bright and bouncy, and it turns out that it's eating nicely on its own and growing well – I think it's regurgitating because it's already stuffed to the gills. But I'll take any opportunity to cuddle a kiwi chick the size of a softball. It was adorable. Then I called in to the clinic to pick up some paperwork. I hadn't been into work for six days and it was *wonderful* to see everyone – as exciting as if I'd been on a desert island. And yet I have a very nice family, a whole farm to roam around on and plenty of jobs to get on with. What about the people who live alone, in town, with non-essential jobs?

Wednesday 25 March

I went to work, since it's tricky doing surgery remotely, and found the surgery had all been cancelled. The front door is blocked by a table, and customers stand outside and call for what they want.

Two police officers turned up, asking if we could sell them hand sanitiser – they've been instructed to stock up on the stuff but there's none left in the country. They were hoping we could sell them some teat wipes in the meantime, but since everyone else in the district also wants teat wipes, we have almost none left.

A series of emails arrived during the morning, announcing decreased hours and pay cuts for everyone. Understandable, but not great for morale. We're going to be separated into two teams, which will have no direct contact whatsoever with one another, and we're being urged to postpone all non-emergency calls while simultaneously continuing to do as much work as possible to keep the business afloat. Right.

I went to the supermarket on the way home. There was no flour, no sugar, no milk powder, no pasta, no tinned spaghetti or baked beans. There was, however, a huge toilet paper pyramid beside the dairy section (which was entirely devoid of milk). At the checkout I was asked to put back one of the loaves of bread in my trolley (I had three – in my excitement at seeing *some* food to buy I forgot about the 'two items only' rule). There was a big group of people, all standing carefully two metres apart, on the pavement outside the chemist's waiting for prescriptions. Everything has an excitingly post-apocalyptic sort of feel.

Thursday 26 March (Day 1 of lockdown)

The Department of Conservation has announced that during the lockdown there's to be no checking of traplines or bait stations on public land (although I'd have thought it was the perfect job for self-isolating), and they'd much prefer that no-one does so on private land either. Apparently, the risk of someone falling over in the bush and needing to be rescued is just too great.

Man, that's depressing.

I seem to have different priorities from most people. I remember when I was little thinking that the World Wildlife Fund was *obviously* a much more deserving charity than, say, the Child Cancer Foundation, since the world *obviously* contained far too many people and far too little nature. I still think it. The risk of coronavirus, with a one percent mortality rate, versus the risk of seriously endangered birds being chewed on? Come *on*.

James and I fed out the palm kernel together this afternoon. There's a lovely soft green fuzz of germinating grass all over the farm. And I may have the rotten silage bale in the bull paddock for garden mulch, if I like. I like very much.

Friday 27 March

Amy brought over a twenty-litre bucket of windfall apples for the pigs this morning. (Her own pig doesn't like apples; it prefers carbs. And as she says, who can blame it?) We chatted for a few minutes at a careful distance. Her family is thoroughly enjoying lockdown so far, and Sean and the girls are building an enormous blanket hut in the living room.

Then, after lunch, Diane called by to bring me two Chelsea Winter cookbooks for my birthday, thus completing the set. What a brilliant present! She said that her children fought today until in desperation she sent them both out in opposite directions for a walk, and that she's decided that it's perfectly acceptable, in these troubled times, to have her first wine of the evening at 2 p.m. I don't think I've ever enjoyed talking to Diane so much in my life.

James finished fixing a bit of fence along the creek, I stewed ten kilos of apples, Ellie made a bouquet of paper flowers and Blake practised spear-throwing with a bamboo stake. Highly productive day all round.

Saturday 28 March

I've been on the phone with Aunty Brenda, who assured me that Everything Will Be Okay and We *Will* All Get Through This. I'm not sure why I'm so irritated, when I agree.

It was a lovely, crisp day – you could see every separate fold of every hill. Ellie and I fed out the palm kernel this morning while Blake and James fed out the silage, and we had soup and garlic bread for lunch. Then, in the afternoon, James and I went down to the creek at the back of the farm, where he filled bait stations and I sprayed tradescantia. Again. The bits I got the first time look good and sick – but they also look like they'll recover nicely if given the chance. And the bits I missed don't look any more accessible than they did when I deferred the job last time. Oh, crap. I foresee this is a twice-a-year-for-the-next-ten-years job, with no guarantee of ultimate success. But on the bright side, we didn't meet a single crazed stag.

Sunday 29 March

I just rolled the ute into the clothesline (parked it beside the veggie garden to pitchfork off a load of rotten silage, forgot to put the handbrake on, clothesline now has a nasty lean) and am soothing my nerves with a glass of wine and a Toffee Pop. It's working very well.

Blake came with me to feed out the palm kernel this morning, and talked all the time without stopping. He's had a brilliant idea – when he's old enough to start manufacturing light sabres, he's going to make me one to use as a pruning saw. It'll be so much quicker and more efficient just to laser off those unwanted branches. I can't wait!

The rabbit that lives under the hay barn in the Saddle Paddock, where James leaves the motorbike and the dogs every day when he feeds out, has got so used to the constant traffic that it lies in the gateway with its paws crossed and only gets up and saunters out of the way when you get within two metres.

I talked to Clare this afternoon. She employs ten people and she's spent the week trying to organise them all into new teams and rosters. She's feeling miserable that, just when things with Dan were looking so promising, she can't see him for at least a month. Most people she sees are taking the whole social distancing thing really seriously – with the exception of the 30-odd people she saw during her morning run who were having a party on someone's lawn.

Monday 30 March

First day of the school holidays, so we can temporarily give up on home schooling. Whew. (Slightly concerning that I feel like that about it after only four days ...)

Today was absolutely lovely. I spent most of it pregnancy-testing beef cows out at the coast, with my very favourite farmers, in yards with a view of the sea. There was only one empty cow to be culled, and they didn't like her anyway. I drove back to the clinic drinking thermos coffee and eating peaches, via a very nice dog with an abscess on his side.

I'm on Team Magenta at work, along with Bill, Melissa, Jess and Emma. Jess says she was really pleased to find herself on this team, 'with all the hillbillies'. I'm not entirely sure what she means, but I *think* it's complimentary.

This evening's sunset was perhaps the most beautiful that I've ever seen. There were thunderstorms and showers all around, the light was an unearthly greenish gold and every flower and raindrop glowed against the smudgy purple sky. The garden looked like Fairyland.

*

After tea, Ellie and I watched *About Time*, cuddled up in James's and my bed, while the boys ate ice cream and watched *Dad's Army* reruns. *About Time* may be my absolute favourite movie ever. (Although that's a big call, when you consider *The Princess Bride* and *Four Weddings and a Funeral* and *Fantastic Beasts* and *Stardust*.) Ellie adored it, but afterwards she dissolved into tears about having to grow up and leave us and go away to high school. I pointed out that she should look on the bright side and consider that we may stay at level-four restrictions for so long that she never gets to high school at all. Made her laugh. Whew.

Wednesday 1 April

It was so nice to get outside today after spending all of yesterday in the clinic doing dry-cow consults by phone. Dry-cow consults always leave me limp and exhausted, although yesterday's farmers were all unprecedentedly happy to talk to me. I'm not letting my head swell; after a week of social isolation people are getting to the stage where they'd greet a Jehovah's Witness with cries of delight.

This morning Blake and I fed out the palm kernel and put up four new bait stations, and then carried on into town from the back of the farm to pick up a tonne of meal and get the groceries.

The supermarket was even more surreal and post-apocalyptic than last week. There was a (carefully spaced out) queue at the door, and they were letting in one person at a time, as someone came out. Most things were available, except flour, but almost all of the customers were scurrying around with their heads down and either surgical masks or scarves over their mouths. The mood seems to have gone from let's-be-sensible-and-careful to full-blown terror – maybe because the first three cases in town have just been announced, imported from a wedding ten days ago in the South Island. (Two of the people who've just tested positive work at the other vet clinic in town, which has now been closed for a fortnight. An elderly man I encountered last week – I picked up a plant for Val from his house but declined to go inside on the grounds that we should all be social distancing, and he was patronisingly amused by my concern – just rang me in a panic to check that it wasn't me who was sick, and that I hadn't exposed him to any nasty germs.)

The woman in front of me at the checkout had covered everything but her eyes with her scarf. She stood peering around suspiciously, presumably in case anyone got too close, while her groceries were scanned and put into a trolley. She then decided to move them all back into her original trolley, one at a time, touching every item only by its corners. It didn't seem to occur to her that she was holding everybody else up, or indeed that it was totally unnecessary. Very painful.

When I got back out to the ute Blake was sitting in the sun with all the windows up, sweat pouring down his little face. He explained that he'd had to close the windows to stop flies getting in. I'd like to think he'd have opened them again before passing out from heat exhaustion, but I'm not entirely sure. He recovered quickly once we got moving, looking at himself thoughtfully in the rear-vision mirror for a while before saying, 'Why does my hair look so *good*?'

*

Text message from Clare this afternoon: she couldn't get wholemeal bread or cucumbers at the supermarket. She is obviously much healthier than I am – a lack of wholemeal bread and cucumbers wouldn't bother me one little bit.

Thursday 2 April, 6 a.m.

I've just had the most horrible dream. Not scary – it just made me feel unlikeable and pathetic, and the feeling isn't fading on waking up.

I dreamt that a girl I used to work with – a bright, bubbly, capable, friendly girl whom everyone liked; the heart and soul of any party – called in to the clinic and, amid all the happy greetings and what-have-you-been-doing-with-yourselfs, she skipped me. And I went through a horrible, uncertain period of telling myself I was overreacting and trying to join the conversation, until she'd pretended not to hear me and refused to meet my eye half-a-dozen times and I realised that I wasn't imagining it; she *did* think I was a total loser.

It doesn't sound like much of a nightmare, but it took me right back to an incident in my first year of university, when I hadn't found a particular group of friends yet and was wondering if there was something wrong with me, and a girl in my halls of residence confirmed it by telling me that she was a really lovely person and usually found it no trouble at all to be nice to absolutely everyone, but for some reason something about me annoyed her so much that she couldn't even force herself to be civil. No offence intended, of course. Don't take it personally, will you?

Hopefully, she's now a miserable person and no-one likes her.

9 p.m.

I found a perfect mushroom ring in the Ridge Paddock this morning, while checking a stoat trap on my way out to shovel palm kernel. I rang home, thinking that mushroom hunting would be a nice expedition for the kids, and Blake arrived ten minutes later on his motorbike. He leapt off his bike, actually standing on a mushroom, but couldn't see any until I went down to show him. He watched me pick them, said he hadn't brought a container so perhaps I should take them along with me, and roared off home again. Hmm.

One of the heifers, due to calve in July, calved this morning instead. Very cute little calf, but what a stuff-up. After racking his brains for some time, and wondering if immaculate conception might actually have occurred, James dimly remembered finding a heifer over the fence from her friends one morning, long ago. He thought no more about it at the time, but maybe she jumped *two* fences, into the neighbours', and they chased her back through the gate in the boundary fence without mentioning it.

Friday 3 April

I can now manoeuvre the front-end loader bucket as I drive, like a professional, rather than stopping the tractor every time I need to lift it up or down. I'm unspeakably proud of myself.

We went on a family expedition to the waterwheel at the back of the farm this afternoon. James fixed the pump, I sprayed tradescantia, the kids climbed waterfalls and the dogs lay in the creek. Then we shifted a mob of ewes on the way home.

We discovered, while making dinner, that the fridge was dead and obviously had been all day. In hindsight, that probably explains the mysterious blowing of a fuse in the kitchen last night. Luckily Val has two fridges, and she emptied one for us, bless her. We went up after dinner to get it, and Thomas and Diane came over too. We had a very nice, somewhat surreal family catch-up, with Val and Trevor on the deck, Thomas and Diane's family on one side of the lawn and us on the other. Then we loaded up the fridge and bore it home on the motorbike trailer.

The neighbours who gave us the calves flagged us down as we passed their house, and rushed out with a bag full of DVDs for the kids. They are so lovely.

Saturday 4 April, 4 p.m.

Today I have:

- Got up early to write (James got up ten minutes later, tried to talk to me and gave up with the comment that yes, he *can* see I'm busy, but if he waited until I wasn't doing something more important, we'd never actually speak at all. Oops.)
- Fed out palm kernel to eleven mobs of heifers
- Cleaned the house
- Made bread with the last remaining flour in the house, if not the country
- Re-potted a tray of baby red-hot pokers
- Moved a large hydrangea across the garden
- Packaged 15 kilos of possum bait into 200-gram bags
- Pruned a dozen trees down behind the dog kennels

Then I sliced the top of my finger with the pruning saw, retreated inside for a plaster and realised I was really, really tired, and that I've slipped into a familiar mental groove. In this groove, I never think: *Goodness, I've accomplished a lot today. How satisfying.* I think: *Huh. Look at that. You can get quite a lot done when you put your back into it; why don't you do it more often, you lazy shit?*

I get a lot done in not-good-enough mode, but it really isn't a happy place to be. And I do know, although I forget, that life is all about the journey, not the destination/people on their deathbeds never wish they'd spent less quality time with their families/[insert platitude of choice here].

Right. I don't actually *have* to spray jasmine, stew apples, mow the lawn, make tea and write 1000 words before bedtime. Instead I will sit down and read *The Quiet Gentleman* for the twenty-sixth or so time, and when my family comes home (James and Blake are down the farm and Ellie is talking to her best friend on the phone), I will *talk to them*.

Val just rang – Trevor is experimenting in the kitchen and has made enough biryani to feed at least a dozen people. How about we come and get some for dinner?

Hooray! The universe is endorsing my decision to rest.

Monday 6 April

I had a text message from Dan this morning, asking if we could please invoice him for grazing. Found the invoice book and discovered that we are, as usual, three months behind. We're all about razor-sharp business principles around here, that's for sure.

I dropped the invoice in his mailbox on the way to work. Dan was on his way home for breakfast, and stopped to talk for a couple of minutes. He says that, two weeks in, he's quite enjoying the lockdown; he's not very sociable and seldom feels like going out, and he always feels guilty about being such a hermit. Now he *can't* be sociable, and it's a great weight off his mind. He also told me, with unprecedented candour, that he and Clare have started handwriting each other letters. They photograph the letters and email them to one another. Neither of them has ever started a relationship by really getting to know the other person, and they're hopeful that it will be a big improvement.

I found this so touching that I'd have hugged him if it weren't for social distancing. Another coronavirus silver lining for him because he would have hated that.

I pregnancy-tested a mob of fat, unpleasant beef cows today. I've never met such uncooperative animals. They wouldn't walk up the race, they waddled backwards at high speed as I tried to insert the probe, they were so far pregnant I had to check lots of them manually, they'd been eating standing hay so that their poo was the consistency of concrete ... It was a herd we haven't scanned before and I was hoping to dazzle the farmer with my efficiency and skill, but I fear that didn't happen.

A young man rang to ask what we could do for a puppy that had been traumatised by fear. They put it outside in its kennel last night just before a thunderstorm (lucky bastards; I wish *we'd* had a thunderstorm), and this morning it was all sad and flat. I asked him to bring it in, and Bill discovered that it was as white as a sheet. He diagnosed rat bait, however, not terror. We dosed the puppy with vitamin K and sent him home with instructions to let him sleep inside and eat plenty of soft food until he was better.

Melissa's small, bad-but-cute dog pooed under my desk. Again. It's very disconcerting to stretch your sock-clad feet out under your desk and encounter a steaming turd. When applied to, Melissa said that her baby would never do such a thing and it must have been some other dog. A startling claim, considering that we're in lockdown and the clinic is not exactly riddled with wandering dogs. When a second poo came to light in the stationery cupboard, she changed tack and said the poor animal must have an upset tummy. If that dog was a child, Melissa would be the sort of mother who says that little Johnny *isn't* a bully; he only hits the other children because he's so sensitive. But on the other hand, Melissa has given me many dozens of fresh eggs. We're all entitled to our blind spots.

Tuesday 7 April

The owner of yesterday's rat bait puppy called this morning to say that the puppy had eaten seven tins of jelly meat and was found out of its box careening around the lounge at midnight. Nice.

In the afternoon I pregnancy-tested a herd of beef cows. Unlike yesterday's mob, they walked nicely up the race and stood still while I scanned them. It made a lovely contrast. I was helped by the farmer's youngest son, a very nice little boy in Blake's class who trotted up and down the boardwalk spraying the empties. He couldn't grasp the concept of social distancing, and mostly wanted to stand on my feet. I spent the first twenty minutes of the job fending him off with the scanner probe before giving up and deciding that as long as I didn't lick the child it would probably be okay.

When I got back to the ute I found four voice messages on my phone. They were as follows:

Blake: *When will you be home?*
Blake: *When will you be home?*
Blake: *Will you be home soon?*
Blake (very plaintive): *Oh, never mind.*

I called him back, and he said that Dad and Ellie had gone down the farm. His life was blighted because he found a hat – a brand-new, extremely cool hat – and James said he could have it but then remembered he'd already promised it to Ellie. I tried to cheer him up, but in vain.

At bedtime he was still dwelling on the hat (which is too big even for me, and makes him look like a mushroom). In desperation I asked him to list three nice things that had happened today. After a long pause, he said, 'Well, I thought I had a hat, for a little while.'

Ellie and I have started watching *Pride and Prejudice*, the six-part BBC version with Colin Firth and Jennifer Ehle, before bed. It's so good.

Wednesday 8 April

Very, very windy. It's amazing how aware you become of wind when you're shovelling a tonne of extremely dusty palm kernel a day. That stuff gets *everywhere*.

James came past on the tractor as I loaded the ute and drew my attention to a large lump of concrete, formerly part of the fertiliser bin wall, that I had broken off and added to my load. I didn't even notice. I may have congratulated myself on my awesome front-end loader technique a little too soon.

Thursday 9 April

A podcast James was listening to today told him that the best indicator of how active and mobile a person will be at 90 is how easily they can sit down on the floor, cross-legged, without putting out a hand to steady themselves, and then stand up again the same way. He tried it, and collapsed in an ungainly heap. I tried it and did it. James was shocked and depressed. We decided the difference must be that I do Pilates and he doesn't, and scheduled a family after-dinner class on the spot.

We had a 35-second thunder shower at lunchtime, long enough to wet the washing I had absent-mindedly left on the lawn but not long enough to wet the grass. Ellie and I seized it as an excuse to stay inside and watch two episodes of *Pride and Prejudice* (which Blake calls *Pride and Poo*) while the boys went mustering, and then Ellie applied herself to the Lego mansion she is building and I went out to fill bait stations.

I had a lovely time – the bush is full of birds, and it was perfect walking weather: cloudy and cold, with an iron-grey sky and gleams of acidy yellow sunshine.

The family Pilates class went well, after we'd banished Blake to the far side of the lounge for farting, giggling and creating a nuisance. We plan to repeat every other day, alternating with planking, and confidently expect to all have abs of steel by the end of the month. They might be quite well covered, though – my darling mother-in-law gave me a bag of flour yesterday and this morning I made a caramel apple cake, containing 300 grams of butter and a whole tin of condensed milk. A third of it has gone already.

Friday 10 April

It's Good Friday today, and seeing as I now have a little flour, I made hot cross buns – half of them glazed and half naked, because Ellie doesn't like glaze and Blake loves it.

On the way home around the road from my palm kernel circuit, I met a local farmer heading home on his side-by-side. He had his smallest two grandchildren with him – at least, I assume he did. All I could see of them was two little tufts of duck fluff sticking up over the dashboard. It was almost unbearably cute.

After lunch we went out to vaccinate, drench and ear-tag the ewe lambs. Miraculously, about two-thirds of them are over 40 kilograms, big enough to go to the ram.

Blake was unusually helpful. He bustled around loading the tags, drafting and chasing lambs up the race. Ellie, on the other hand, lurked sourly at the back of the pen, scowling and muttering and making faces at her brother when she thought we weren't looking. I've noticed this phenomenon before; the sweeter and more charming one child is, the worse the other behaves.

Saturday 11 April

School holidays are officially over after Easter, and the kids' online learning programs arrived this morning via email. They have daily lessons and weekly projects, which are to be uploaded to their respective Google classrooms when completed. It all looks very professional – the schedules made my heart sink, and I'm not even the one who has to follow them. I'll have to oversee the process, though, so I'd better dredge up some enthusiasm. We cannot, after all, just continue to use the children as domestic servants and gate openers indefinitely.

This afternoon I finished filling the bait stations around the main block of bush (a tomtit followed me and supervised) while James brought up the ewes and cut five rams out to go with the hoggets. Then Blake and I loaded the rams onto the back of the ute and delivered them to their new teenage girlfriends while James and Ellie put the ewes back.

The rams were most enthusiastic about meeting the hoggets. I hope this was because the ewes are already all pregnant and they were bored rather than because they prefer innocent and nubile girls to older women.

Sunday 12 April

Ellie returned from a trip to see the pet sheep that live below the woolshed this afternoon with a gift pack from Amy containing a dozen tiny Easter eggs, pictures and letters from each of her little girls and two full bread bags of flour. Amy is wonderful.

Our regular Pilates classes, I regret to admit, have been deferred for the last two evenings. Instead we have lolled on the couch watching *Aladdin*, which we bought for the kids on Google Play as a token of appreciation for much farm work and vacuuming.

Monday 13 April

In a burst of enthusiasm, I have started writing a book about a princess, who is kidnapped by very inept revolutionaries, and a family of goose farmers who live in a swamp. It's a sort of fairy tale, and I want it to be funny and charming and evocative and sweet and uplifting. Stories never come out as funny and charming and evocative and sweet and uplifting on paper as they were in my head, but it's a good aim. I don't imagine the market for adult fairy tales about princesses finding happiness in swamps is very large, but never mind. You can't go around writing books in the expectation that they'll start bidding wars and become international bestsellers. The only way to remain even vaguely sane is to tell yourself firmly that you're doing it for fun, and any interest in anything you've written by anyone at all is an unexpected bonus.

Tuesday 14 April

A quiet day at work today. I spent it scanning bits of paper to comply with new legal requirements and saving them onto dairy farmers' files on the computer. I don't understand how compiling lists of the drugs farmers have on hand at the time of their milk quality consults is going to improve animal health or prevent drug residues in milk, or why printouts of restricted veterinary medicines now have to be countersigned by both farmer and vet, but mine is not to reason why.

A bright spot among the meaningless paperwork was a discussion about annoying after-hours calls. Bill, I think, has the most recent winner – he drove almost all the way to Hamilton a few months ago at eleven o'clock on Sunday night to put down a goat that had been near death for several weeks. Then the owner complained that he was a bit gruff, and not as sweet and sympathetic as she'd have liked.

My latest total waste of time was driving for an hour and a quarter one Saturday afternoon to see a dribbling 700-kilogram steer on a lifestyle block without a single stock-proof fence. We spent an hour trying (fruitlessly) to encourage the steer to enter and then remain in a yard made of two pallets and a broken gate, while the steer's owners said plaintively, 'Why don't you have a dart gun or something?'

After work I went to the supermarket. I was unloading my groceries onto the conveyor when the girl serving me said, 'You're actually over the limit on some of these items.'

'Oh!' I said. 'Sorry. I didn't think there were restrictions still.'

'Just on some things. Like tins – you've got two of spaghetti and one of baked beans, and the limit is two in total.'

'Well, I can put some back.'

'No, that's okay, I'm just telling you for next time. You can only have one block of cheese and just two tins of fruit. But I've put them through this time.'

'Why don't you put up signs so people know?'

'Look, it's okay, I'm just letting you know for next time. You're allowed *four* different bottles of alcohol now.'

'How is anyone supposed to know that if there aren't any signs?'

'There are signs,' she said vaguely. (There weren't.) 'And it comes over the sound system.' (The sound system wasn't on.) 'There's no need to get upset.'

'I'm not upset!' I said. (I was.) 'But if there are no signs telling me, I'm going to keep taking too many things, and I expect everyone else will too.'

'No, *most* people are very reasonable. Look, don't worry, I'm just *telling* you …'

Anyway, I got my three tins of peaches, two tins of spaghetti and one of baked beans, and a bag of grated Edam as well as a block of tasty cheese. I'm such a selfish and unreasonable food hoarder.

Wednesday 15 April

Thirty mil of rain overnight. Thank the lord. Shovelled my palm kernel in a howling gale, and am now feeling thoroughly exfoliated.

The kids have watched *Aladdin* six times in the last three days. It's a lovely movie, wonderfully choreographed, but the songs are starting to run through my head on a sort of constant loop.

Thursday 16 April

More rain – yay! – and the cattle have turned the ground around each palm kernel trough to mud. Stopping the ute alongside involves lining it up and sliding the last metre or two, which gives me a pleasant boy-racer-ish feeling. Sometimes I get it wrong and slide right into the side of a concrete trough, but who cares? The ute is 30 years old and a couple more dents to the doors are neither here nor there. My grandfather, I recall, drove his Land Rover like that. The brakes weren't very good and the tyres were pretty iffy, so he just drove it at the nearest bank when he wanted to stop. Good man.

I was listening, as I slithered around the farm, to an earnest American podcast about the importance of maintaining our social connections mid-pandemic. It inspired me to ring my mother, who said, 'Oh, hello, darling. All well? Must go; I've got Miriam on the other line.'

I tried Suzanne next, and we chatted for about a minute before one of her children started hitting the other over the head with a wooden cow and she had to go. Oh well, at least I tried.

I did achieve some meaningful social connection, however. I was picking mushrooms beside the road gate when a very nice local contractor arrived on a tractor (he's going to under-sow a couple of hay paddocks for us). He promptly leapt off his tractor and enfolded me in a warm hug, which was very sweet but slightly alarming, in these times of physical distancing.

Ellie, model child, did her schoolwork and made soup for lunch while the rest of us were out. After lunch I asked Blake to start his schoolwork, and went outside to plant out some seedlings. Blake appeared five minutes later and practised jumping off the roof like Aladdin. On being asked to do some work he announced he would do a project on his favourite tree, and climbed to the top of it in the name of research. I accompanied him inside, where he sobbed pitifully and wrote:

My favrit tree is a silver Berch. JJ and me pertended it was a ship. The branchs are in the right place for my feet.

I suggested he do a little research to round out his project; he borrowed my phone for the purpose and added:

They come from Erope and Asia.

Hmm.

Friday 17 April

I don't like jelly. Never did. Can't imagine I ever will. It's the way it slithers down your throat before your tongue and teeth have time to do anything about it.

Last week Blake and Ellie both made jelly. Both offered me some multiple times, until in desperation I cried, '*I don't like jelly!* What part of this do you turkeys not understand?'

There was a short pause, and then Ellie said, 'So would you like some jelly *now*?' and she, Blake and James all collapsed into hysterical laughter.

The new standard reply to any maternal or wifely request in this house is, 'No thanks, but would you like some jelly?'

Things are feeling a bit Groundhog Day-ish around here, after three and a bit weeks of lockdown. Housework, schoolwork, farm work, lunch, more farm work, TV (especially *Outback Wrangler* – we can happily watch people catch huge crocodiles for hours on end), dinner, reading, bed. Over and over and over. Today was varied by finding a beautiful mushroom ring in the Flax Dam Paddock, and discovering that Blake had put away the washing by stuffing it, unfolded, into the linen cupboard. Also by cutting a water pipe with the spade while transplanting half-a-dozen lacebark seedlings that came up in the garden just outside the front door. James was very nice about it.

'What are we doing tomorrow?' Ellie asked when I went to kiss her goodnight. My list of potential exciting activities was:

- Check stoat traps
- Mulch garden with rotten silage
- Read aloud
- Make apple crumble
- Make paper flowers to stick on the dining room windows to prevent birds flying into them
- Write to Aunty Sue

She was unenthused.

Saturday 18 April

We went for a family mushroom-hunting expedition this afternoon, between showers. It was a beautiful afternoon, all golden and sparkly, with curls of mist smoking up off the bush in the gullies. We were in the ram paddock beside the woolshed when Thomas, Diane, Rachel and Holly came past, heading down the road on a walk. Thomas and Diane were walking hand in hand. Of course, they disengaged instantly on seeing us (both James and Thomas think that holding your wife's hand in public denotes a shameful weakness of character), but how lovely. So nice to be reminded that the story I've been telling myself about Thomas nobly hiding his broken heart for the last seventeen years, since first he saw me across a crowded cattle yard, is made up. Real life doesn't work like that. Thank goodness.

Our three resident quail have finished the seed bell and are now wandering moodily around the lawn, waiting for the next handout and picking on the sparrows rather than foraging for themselves. Is this an illustration of what the welfare system does to people? (Not that I think we shouldn't have a welfare system; people starving in the gutters is such a bad look for a country.)

The four weeks of nationwide level-four lockdown finishes in a few days. I wonder what they'll revise it to? There was an opinion piece in the news today saying the lockdown was totally over the top and has done untold damage to the economy – after all, we've only had eleven deaths to date, all of them elderly people with existing respiratory issues. It doesn't seem to have occurred to the genius writing this piece that the rapidly decreasing infection rate is the *result* of the lockdown, not a sign that the whole thing was unnecessary. Unless, of course, the article was designed to stir us all up into righteous indignation and defence of the government's security measures ... What a delightfully conspiracy theory-ish thought.

Monday 20 April

It's been announced that level-four restrictions will continue another week, just to make sure we don't get community transmission of the virus when we start expanding our bubbles. Fair enough.

Ellie's home-learning pack from the Ministry of Education has arrived, and it's *awesome*. She has a couple of really great workbooks, two school journals, a little book about the history of Kawhia Harbour, a bendy ruler, a packet of colouring pencils and a couple of pens. She's very excited and has already done the first week's work. Her teacher has also implemented daily Google meetings and got the whole class learning the language of their choice. I can't see why we'd ever send her back to school – not only does she seem to be learning more at home but she does most of the housework and makes a mean cheese scone.

Today at work we had no fewer than three dogs with upset stomachs. One of them, a very nice bull terrier with a doting owner, visited twice during the day and then went to another practice for further work-up because the owner was concerned the dog wasn't recovering quickly enough. The diagnosis at the other practice was the same as ours: if you give a dog with a nasty allergy to beef a packet of mince when you run out of his normal food, he's going to have a pretty sore tummy for a couple of days – even if it *was* really good-quality mince.

Tuesday 21 April

We suddenly realised today that Bill's last-ever day of work is almost here, and we can't have our planned leaving party for him. The new plan is to have a socially distant pot-luck lunch for him on his last day. We'll make all his favourite foods — cucumber sandwiches, boiled fruit cake, chicken drumsticks, sausage rolls and savoury scones. Absolutely no garlic. (We checked with his family.) The gift, if it can be sourced during current restrictions, will be an amazing tow-behind-the-lawnmower tip-trailer, filled with dark beer, liquorice and other delicious things.

I don't know what we'll do without Bill. He can wrangle the nastiest cats and make a cast for a cow's broken leg out of silage tape and electric fence standards. He has an infinite number of cool stories and is the only person in the building willing to perform minor surgery on his colleagues. He's also one of the nicest people on the planet.

I was late home tonight. A woman who desperately needed an Animal Health Plan for her meatworks audit — but had been far too busy for the last two days to return my calls requesting information so I could write it — rang at 4.45 p.m. She gave me her lambing and shearing dates and told me kindly that she didn't need the plan until tomorrow, so I could do it in the morning if I wanted to. Since I'm not working tomorrow and have many, many better things to do than writing her stinking health plan, I thought I'd rather just get it over with. It took me an hour, and when I'd emailed it to her and went to charge it out, the computer wouldn't let me overwrite the standard fee, so

I was forced to charge $95 rather than the $200 I felt was only right and just.

I had a text message from James saying, *Let me know when you're leaving*. I did, and got home to a piping-hot plate of steak, mushrooms, potato cake and cauliflower cheese, flanked by a glass of chilled Sauvignon. Totally restored my good mood.

Wednesday 22 April

I made a proper boiled fruitcake for Bill's leaving lunch today. It was quite an involved exercise, involving a trip to town for fruit, a trip to Cafe Val for flour, and a second trip to Val (Blake went on his bike) to borrow the special wooden Christmas cake tin. I finally got it into the oven and went out spraying, leaving Ellie to watch it. When I returned, the cake was sitting on the bench, its top charred and blackened. I didn't even have the consolation of being able to blame Ellie – I set the timer for two hours and asked her to check it at fifteen-minute intervals thereafter, and it was burnt when the timer first went off.

Well, it could be worse. We have enough dried fruit – just – to make another one, and after trimming the edges there's quite a decent amount of unburnt cake left for us.

We came back from spraying with a goat. As you do. Blake and I heard it bleating from behind a gorse bush across the creek in the neighbour's back paddock – it popped its head out, Blake took a step forwards, the goat took a step forwards, and they spent the next two hours exploring hand in hoof while I sprayed. The goat accompanied us back up the hill to the four-by-four. Blake looked at me with eyes of hope. I said, 'Well, see if it will sit in the footwell, then.' It hopped up, laid its chin on my accelerator foot and went to sleep.

Its name is Gaston. It's small and caramel-coloured, with big soft eyes and a heart-shaped white spot on its forehead. Tomorrow we plan to drench it (it's skinny and pot-bellied, and I'm sure it's riddled with worms) and castrate it.

I can't believe we now have a goat. It's a well-known fact that goats are only happy when:

1. Eating the wiring off your tractor
2. Breaking into your house and jumping on your bed
3. Ring-barking your fruit trees
4. Eating your favourite rhododendron and then collapsing in agony with stomach cramps

These are not made-up examples – I have personally witnessed every single one of them in goats belonging to close friends and colleagues.

But the damn thing is adorable, so we'll just have to put up with it. Now we just need a possum, a stoat and a magpie, and we'll have the full set of pest species.

Thursday 23 April

It's really, properly autumn now. The poplars are golden and the grass is luminous green, netted all over with fine spider webs. There are mushroom rings and coprosma berries and birds everywhere. The crabapple on the lawn is bright scarlet and the kids have started feeding sugar water to the tuis and bellbirds.

In the gravel in front of the house, all the special oxalis bulbs my aunt gave me have put up tiny leaves and little silky flowers. There are patches of shiny yellow, pale pink, hot pink, salmon and mauve. Some have bright green clover-like leaves, some have little flat furry fans, some are spotted or burgundy. The autumn crocuses are out, and the cyclamen, and the nerines. There's something extra special about autumn flowers – they're so pure and clear and delicate.

We castrated, drenched and vaccinated Gaston the goat this morning. He didn't seem particularly perturbed by any of it (perhaps the amount of pain relief I gave him had something to do with that) and is now cruising around in the pig paddock, graciously accepting apples, carrots and marshmallows from the children.

James mentioned today in passing that one of his happiest memories is going on a school trip, aged five. He has no idea where they went or what they saw, but vividly remembers going to the bakery in town and being given his first custard square. I made him some at lunchtime (the Edmonds cookbook recipe is excellent, especially if you double the quantity of custard) and have thus guaranteed lifelong gratitude and devotion. Well, weeklong, at least, probably. Certainly until bedtime.

Friday 24 April

Blake's school pack arrived today in the mail. He was beside himself with excitement and leapt right into action. He made a mistake, in pen, on the first question, and wept tears of bitter despair because now his nice clean book was ruined and there was no point in doing any more, ever.

I was in a lousy mood this afternoon. James decided to come and check the stoat traps with me, which should have warmed my heart but didn't. We all went, and I stalked along, sighing audibly every time Blake stopped (approximately every seven seconds) and generally being a blight on a pleasant family outing. Eventually James enquired whether I felt he should be fencing or spraying gorse rather than frittering away time with his family. I did. Not cool. I hate this sick, guilty feeling that creeps up on me and tells me that any moment not spent working is a moment wasted. It's so bloody joyless and puritanical.

Sunday 26 April

Lounged around the house drinking coffee and reading *The Other Wind* this morning, thus losing forever an hour that could have been spent working. Felt I'd struck a major blow against my puritanical tendencies.

Discovered yet again that remembering to disengage the handbrake on the tractor does wonders for the smoothness of my take-offs.

Picked up chestnuts for the pigs with Blake – or to be truly accurate, I picked up chestnuts for the pigs and he picked up chestnuts to throw at fence posts.

*

I was standing naked in the kitchen this afternoon, clutching a big Waikato beer bottle, when James got home. He was very sceptical about my entirely reasonable explanation that I was on the way to the shower, hot and thirsty after mowing the lawn, and had paused for a drink of kombucha, which I decanted this morning into beer bottles to store in the fridge.

Favourite coronavirus meme to date: a picture of the trikini, with top, bottoms and face mask all in pretty floral Lycra.

Monday 27 April

I have been listening to Blake reading aloud, which is an exercise in extreme frustration. He reads flawlessly when he concentrates, but 90 percent of the time he just glances at the page, picks a word at random and makes a wild stab at the rest of the sentence. This ensures that what he reads makes no sense whatsoever. And reading gibberish is boring, so his mind wanders, and instead of reading the next sentence properly he just picks a word at random …

When we went out to feed the dogs and give the goat and pigs a bedtime snack, there were half-a-dozen native snails on the lawn. Their shells are glossy brown and about the size of my little fingernail, and lie flat across their electric blue bodies. We never used to see any until we started trapping rats and hedgehogs. According to Google there are about 1400 species of native slugs and snails. Most are carnivorous, almost all are endangered and only about half have been officially described. Maybe these ones are completely unknown to science.

Tuesday 28 April

Today the nation has moved to level three, which means that we can go through the McDonald's drive-through and enlarge our bubbles (slightly, if we really, really need to). In a shock move, Val and Trevor have joined Trevor's sister's bubble, not Thomas and Diane's. Diane is deeply put out. I think she was looking forward to her children spending most of their time at Nana's.

Wednesday 29 April

It was Bill's last day today, and he spent the morning spaying Jess's very beloved old dog, a job that was surely in the running for Most Stressful Procedure in the World. The only slight consolation was that if anything went wrong (which of course it didn't), he was leaving anyway. We had a very nice lunch, his present arrived in time and Sophie, who is a millennial and thus can make a computer do anything she wants, made him a really cool card, but it was still miserable to be saying goodbye.

Friday 1 May

As I lay dozing in bed this morning, I had a small epiphany. The answer to my nagging concerns about the dullness and sameness of this diary is obvious! I'll write about how I'm currently travelling in England! All *sorts* of exciting things have been happening – going to a new school, the midnight swims in that amazing swimming pool with magnetic walls so the water looks like it's been cut off with a knife, the fire, the baby … I can't imagine why I thought I should pretend I was still at home.

At which point I woke up properly and realised that, no, I'm *not* in the south of England on a school exchange with Ellie's teacher, my cousin Amanda and neighbour Dan. (Why them? The subconscious mind is a strange, strange thing.) And yet it was all so plausible ten minutes ago.

Actual, rather than imaginary, schooling is going pretty well. Ellie quietly gets out her work every morning and gets on with it; Blake starts with bitter complaint and moves through despair, grudging compliance, interest, excitement and pride in a job well done. The whole process seems a bit exhausting to me, but he seems to enjoy the emotional variety.

James found another rotten silage bale today. He dropped it on the back of the ute for me after I'd finished feeding palm kernel and I brought it home. I couldn't spend the afternoon with it because we drenched two mobs of calves, but it's waiting for me on the lawn, and I can hardly wait for morning to start spreading it. Which is lucky, since I have to get it off the back of the ute before I can feed out.

Saturday 2 May

Dan took his heifers home today and brought his calves over. He and James drenched them, and then James ran them down the hill towards their new paddock. At the first crossing Taz the huntaway, whose enthusiasm greatly exceeds his intelligence, barked, and four of the calves leapt in panic off the crossing into a deep swamp. Three of the four paddled over to the bank and climbed out. The fourth crawled under a willow tree and had hysterics. James took off his boots, joined her beneath the willow tree and chased her out, whereupon she took three wavering steps along the bank before jumping back into an even deeper and less accessible bit of swamp.

At that point James rang me and I came down with the ute and my long cow-casting rope. We dropped a loop over the calf's head and towed her, with no cooperation from her at all, out onto the bank. She then leapt to her feet and made a spirited attempt to strangle herself on the end of the rope. We got her free eventually, but not until she'd covered us both with mud. Tiresome, but at least she weighed 250 kilograms rather than 500.

Sunday 3 May

James brought the ewes up to the woolshed to draft out the rams and drench the thin ones. Three-quarters of them were thin – not appallingly, welfare-concern thin, but thinner than the nice, plump condition you want them to be at mating time – and the mood in the shed was one of snappishness and gloom.

I got Blake to collect some faecal samples as we ran them through, to see whether worms were part of the problem or if it was just straight underfeeding. He took his job very seriously, and stood watching like a hawk in the back pen. Every time a ewe lifted her tail he was there, pottle in hand.

It rained steadily all afternoon, which was lovely. Gaston the goat did not agree, and at 8 p.m. he arrived at the back door, crying broken-heartedly. Ellie took him back to his little house and fed him bits of apple and tucked him up, and then lay awake worrying about him and wondering if she should take a sleeping bag down the paddock to be with him.

Monday 4 May

Gaston stayed in his paddock all night and greeted Ellie cheerfully when she rushed out at the crack of dawn to see him. Thank goodness, because if he decides that fences are for losers and starts to wander at will through the garden eating rhododendrons and ringbarking apple trees he'll have to be tied up, and that's just miserable.

Work was pretty quiet today. A huntaway came in at lunchtime with a possible uterine infection. She was on heat last week, not eating and had, perhaps, a very slight swelling in her caudal abdomen. But only very slight, and she has no fever. I filled her up with antibiotics and anti-inflammatories and she started eating, although not with wild enthusiasm. I have a feeling we'll have to spay her tomorrow.

The faecal samples from our ewes showed only a few worm eggs, which was good, because they aren't infested with worms, but bad, because we obviously haven't fed them as well as we thought we had. Droughts suck.

I had a moment of concern, this evening, worried that I'm completely out of touch with current events and contemporary pop culture. I haven't looked at the news for days or Facebook for weeks, and have seen no TV except *Aladdin* and *Outback Wrangler*. So I sat down with my phone to bring myself up to date. An hour later I emerged from a random internet spiral that included: the prime minister's championship of New Zealand fashion; a very cool lady who's started posting cooking videos on YouTube and has a tendency to drop her phone into pots of mince in moments of excitement; concern that the government may short-circuit the *Resource Management Act* and approve all sorts of ecologically dodgy projects in an attempt to kickstart the economy; an author I know starting a podcast; and a long list of TV shows everyone is talking about but which I'd never heard of. I now feel dazed, and have a nasty sinking feeling that everyone else in the country (actually, everyone else in the world) is doing something marvellously creative during lockdown while I shovel palm kernel, supervise schoolwork and eat too much cake.

Tuesday 5 May

After dreaming all night about spaying dogs with uterine infections, I got to work and found the sick huntaway leaping around in her kennel. She pranced beside me when I took her out, and then inhaled her breakfast without bothering to chew it. So she's gone home on antibiotics, even though I'm not entirely sure what infection I'm treating, or even if one exists. This is not the sort of approach that impresses advocates of responsible antibiotic use – but on the other hand her owners live miles out of town and will be understandably pissed off if she suffers a relapse.

We spent the morning drying off a herd. The vets don't usually do much drying off; it's organised by the vet technicians, and they have teams of casual staff to help, mostly farmers' wives. But this year, thanks to coronavirus and social distancing, we've been conscripted. It's the same sort of job as security guarding – mostly boring, but occasionally fraught with peril. The cows are milked just before we arrive, and then rowed up again in the cowshed. Aproned and gloved, with shin pads on our forearms as protection from being kicked, we scrub the end of every teat with alcohol wipes and insert tubes of long-acting antibiotic, to stop them getting mastitis between drying off and calving next spring. Between cows we disinfect and dry our hands, and after each row we put on new gloves. Every person carries a different-coloured can of spray paint and marks each cow they treat. I can now add a new worry to an already long list – someone ringing up and saying, 'Seventeen cows with blue dots have horrible mastitis. What moron was blue?'

Today's cows were angelically quiet, and it all went smoothly. And as a bonus, I discovered that the bags of dry cow antibiotic are held shut with cable ties *that can be released and reused!* They'll make the best plant ties *ever*. Nobody else seemed to share my enthusiasm for adjustable cable ties, so I came home with a dozen. The moral of this story is that small things can lead to great happiness. (Unless the moral is that simple-minded people are easily pleased.)

One of Ellie's friends sent us a link to Messenger Kids, which allows Ellie to set up her own Messenger account and message her friends from my phone. It also allows her to send me messages and cute stickers, which is lovely, except that passing my cell phone back and forth so we can write messages to one another does seem ever so slightly inefficient ...

Wednesday 6 May

Bubbles the pig has got rid of one of her nose rings and is ploughing the paddock with great enthusiasm. Gaston the goat was standing on the driveway this morning. James's method of dealing with these disasters was to tell me firmly that something would have to be done and then go down the farm. My strategy so far has been to earnestly agree with him. There are pros and cons to this approach. The biggest pro is that neither of us has actually had to do anything. The major con, of course, is that nothing has been done. Oh well. Perhaps the goat will decide that it's better to stay home and the pig that digging is overrated. You never know.

We spent a pleasant hour planting trees this afternoon, on a siding James fenced off a few months ago when he was fixing a section of fence around the edge of the bush. We had about 50 native trees, which seemed like a lot when I bought them last week but looked very sparse when planted. Still, it's a start.

After dinner, in a burst of helpfulness, Blake emptied the dishwasher. Unfortunately, the dishes had not yet been washed. You'd have thought he might have noticed as he slung knives smeared with peanut butter and coffee-stained mugs into the drawers, but no.

Thursday 7 May

The temperature dropped to two degrees last night, and a bank of cold, grey cloud rolled in at dawn to keep the cold in.

Today's achievements:

- Folded two loads of washing
- Vacuumed

- Made a pot roast, a loaf of sourdough bread and a batch of chocolate peppermint slice
- Helped Blake edit a story about trolls and portals and buffalo-eating tigers
- Fed out palm kernel
- Mustered and weighed lambs (most of the little dears are now big enough to go to the works, thank God)
- Cut bamboo stakes and staked the trees we planted yesterday, so as to find them next summer in the long grass
- Sat in on Ellie's Zoom interview for boarding school next year. (It went well, I think, apart from an awkward moment when the hostel manager asked why Ellie wanted to board. She *doesn't* want to, and the dire state of the local school is the only reason we're even considering it, but saying that probably wouldn't have given the impression of happy anticipation we wished to project.)
- Watched *Thor: Ragnarok*
- Read Blake a chapter of *A Wizard of Earthsea*

After which I wandered into our bedroom, where James was reading in bed, and asked, 'Do you think I look alright?'

This tremulous plea for reassurance was met with a critical look, a deep sigh and, 'We-ell, beggars can't be choosers.'

Some women have partners who pay them compliments, bring them flowers and send them romantic text messages. Mine insults me, brings me dead possums and sends text messages reading, *We need rice.* I've obviously gone horribly wrong somewhere.

However, I beat him with a pillow for a while, and felt much better.

Saturday 9 May

It's been the most beautiful day ever. Crisp, fresh air, soft purple mist, single golden leaves spiralling gently down against the purest, deepest blue skies … We spent the afternoon dagging lambs, and even dagging was a pleasure.

Amy rang this morning to ask me if there are any vaccinations they should be giving their pig. They have given up all thought of eating it – it still sleeps snuggled up with its favourite sheep every night, and whenever one of the children passes the fence it rushes up and smiles at her, crinkling up its little piggy eyes in delight.

There have been either no, one or two cases of coronavirus per day for the last week, nationwide, and we are expecting an imminent announcement that we're moving to level two. From what I understand, level-two life involves very few restrictions, except that we can't travel overseas and shouldn't lick one another. Life is good.

In a brief flicker of enthusiasm for social media, I decided to post a few photos of what we've been doing during lockdown on Facebook. A search through my phone discovered a couple of nice sunsets, some native snails, an enormous knot in Ellie's hair after she neglected to brush it for a week, a series of pictures of the back end of the goat, many screenshots of Taylor Swift and the genie from *Aladdin*, and a very unflattering shot of me shovelling palm kernel. Not really what I was hoping for, sadly.

Monday 11 May

Hooray! We're going down to level two on Thursday. Life will resume more or less as normal, except that we're to remember, as a nation, to please keep washing our hands and not have big parties.

Val responded to the announcement by immediately sending out a family-wide invitation for dinner on Friday night. The children are also invited to stay the night and have a luscious breakfast on Saturday morning. They are wildly excited, and Blake has already packed.

I had a very disconcerting conversation with a man outside the supermarket today. He was at the next checkout to mine, and as I came out of the supermarket he drove past, leant out his window and said, 'I noticed you looking at that woman with all the piercings.'

I'm not sure whether he was agreeing with me that she really did look a sight, or telling me off for judging my fellow human beings, but it was a bit alarming, because I'd honestly scarcely noticed her. I was just standing in the checkout line staring vaguely ahead of me at nothing in particular. Is my habitual expression one of revulsion and disdain?

I assured him I hadn't been looking at her at all, but I don't think he believed me.

Tuesday 12 May

I spent a lovely day out at the coast today. I pregnancy-tested 250 beef cows through very nice yards, assisted by very nice farmers. I had apple and feijoa pie for lunch on the side of the road overlooking the sea, and went on to investigate several sudden deaths in a mob of Angus weaner calves.

The calves were bizarre. They were weaned a month ago and brought in yesterday for drenching, and several of them were all shaky and staggery. They attacked the motorbike and twitched and fell over, and two of them that were drafted out into a paddock by the yards to recover sat down and died. Before they were drenched, not afterwards.

The post-mortem revealed only a long list of things that *hadn't* killed them. They were fat; they'd been eating; they didn't have worms; their livers, kidneys, hearts, lungs and intestines all looked beautiful; no mouth ulcers; nothing but grass in their stomachs. We went for a drive to the back of the farm, to the paddock they'd been in for the last week. Soft green grass, clean water, not a poisonous plant to be seen. One more staggery calf, that considered charging us, ran away and collapsed on a distant hillside, just as described. He wasn't blind, he wasn't in respiratory distress, he was fat and glossy – he just couldn't quite control his legs. So I collected a multitude of post-mortem samples in case anyone else could suggest a useful test, and went away.

Back at the clinic we all agreed that the symptoms suggested a poisoning more than anything else, and Sophie found a description of phalaris staggers – tremors, aggression, hind-limb weakness and occasionally death when stressed – that seemed to fit the bill. I've sent the farmers some pictures of phalaris grass so they can go and look for it in last week's paddock, but I'm not really expecting they'll find any.

All very unsatisfactory, especially for the farmers without a good answer.

Thursday 14 May

I am the front-end loader *queen*. Just saying. You should watch me scoop palm kernel; it's poetry in motion.

Other achievements of note today: I wrote 600 words of my new book; drafted lambs; learnt what homophones are (they're words that sound the same but have different meanings, like *aloud* and *allowed* – *not* musical instruments that only make one sound, like triangles. I still think it was a good guess, though); sprayed privet around the Long Swamp; went for a walk with Ellie and Blake (during which we not only enjoyed the fresh air and autumn colours but practised percentages); dug out an extremely vicious dead rosebush; and transplanted a lacebark tree. I am now feeling revoltingly smug and virtuous.

Blake and I have finished *A Wizard of Earthsea* and started *The Tombs of Atuan*. He's loving the series, and keeps interrupting me as I read to ask in-depth questions about the art of wizardry. I think he's planning to be archmage when he grows up. Reading Ursula K. Le Guin is very humbling when you're trying to write a story about a made-up place – she does it so much better than anyone else, before or since, that you wonder why on earth you'd even try.

Sunday 17 May

Dinner at Val's on Friday night was a wild success. Of course we've all, apart from Thalia and Adam, seen each other in passing over the last two months, but it hasn't been the same. There were actually twelve of us for dinner, and at level two only ten people are supposed to gather together, but we were feeling reckless.

Thalia and Adam found lockdown pretty heavy-going. They're not house-and-garden people at all – they have a huge circle of friends and go away most weekends – and they found walks around the block a poor substitute for weekends in the Coromandel. Thalia, Adam said, developed a terrible habit of video-calling a friend and then putting her phone down in some random spot and wandering off. He said it was very distressing to leap out of the shower and start drying himself, and then notice an appalled face watching him from the corner of the bathroom sink.

'That was only Mum,' Thalia protested. 'She's seen it all before.'

'But not usually from *quite* that angle,' Val murmured, and we all collapsed into hysterical laughter.

The kids had a lovely sleepover. They made an absolutely palatial blanket fort in Val's spare room, with Trevor as consulting structural engineer, and all four of them spent the night in it. On Saturday morning Val cooked each one the cafe-style breakfast of his or her choice (they all wanted something different, so she ended up making crepes, American-style pancakes, omelette and eggs Benedict). When I arrived at lunchtime to pick them up, she told me she'd loved every second of it. Best grandmother *ever*.

*

Clare dropped in briefly this afternoon, on her way back to Auckland. She smiled constantly and appeared to be lost in a happy dream. Halfway through her coffee she suddenly got up and said she'd have to go that instant; it was vitally important that she beat the Auckland traffic. Lies, all lies. I am 99.9 percent sure she went straight back to Dan's place to say goodbye all over again. I'm delighted for them both.

Monday 18 May

A lovely huntaway came in for a mammary gland lump removal. We knocked her out, and I was palpating the edges of the lump to see where my surgical margins should be when I discovered a new, egg-sized lump deep in her armpit. The chance of complete surgical resection of an aggressive mammary cancer that has already spread to the lymph nodes – and probably further – was so low that I just woke her up again.

The poor dog. Chemotherapy really isn't an option for elderly farm dogs. Lucky I'm human.

The kids went back to school today. Blake was delirious with joy; Ellie was resigned.

Tuesday 19 May

Aaghhh! We're shearing on Thursday and Friday, there was no baking powder in the supermarket, I'm on call tonight and working tomorrow, the bills are due, and the end-of-year accounts need to be closed off and delivered to the accountant.

This means my annual grapple with the stock reconciliation is at hand. I don't feel strong enough for any of it.

This morning was appalling. James left at five thirty to dag 1100 ewes for shearing. The kids had to be dragged out of bed, and the ritual of breakfasts and lunches and feeding of multiple pets seemed to take forever. I swept Ellie's beloved ceramic pineapple off her windowsill while opening her curtains and broke it, and I was late to work.

On a lighter note, my current bedtime book is a futuristic novel, written in the 1930s and set in the 70s. The heroine is currently on a plane between London and New York – a plane with a restaurant, individual bedrooms, and both a first-class and second-class lounge. She just had a short nap and splashed her face with refreshing radium water on waking up. Excellent stuff.

Thursday 21 May

I cooked frantically all morning, with a brief outing to the woolshed to look at a hogget that one of the shearers had cut on the leg. James thought he'd missed the hamstring. He hadn't. So James killed her and hung her up. Poor little thing. Oh well, these things happen.

This evening I said in passing that it was a shame about the hogget, but it would be nice to have some lamb in the freezer. Oh no, James said cheerfully, the shearer had asked to buy the lamb and James had said yes. The shearer asked him what he wanted for it, and James said, 'A box of beer.'

A box of beer? The bloke ruins a beautiful in-lamb hogget, worth $120 at the works and considerably more at the sale, and then James sells him the carcass for a $30 box of beer? Heaven give me strength! Generosity is a wonderful trait, but James really does carry it to extremes. And I can't help thinking that someone really decent wouldn't have taken the deal, but would have paid fairly for the lamb, and thrown in a box of beer by way of apology for having been the cause of its premature demise.

Friday 22 May

Yesterday I made bacon-and-egg pie, chocolate cake, lasagne, shepherd's pie, bread, coleslaw, chocolate brownies, ginger crunch, lemon cake, coconut loaf and apple shortcake. After which I never wanted to see the kitchen again. But all I had to do this morning was make another loaf of bread, heat the shepherd's pie and make cheese scones for morning smoko.

I made my scones (using the very last of the butter, milk and cheese) while Blake stood at my elbow telling me there was nothing in the house for him to eat for either breakfast or lunch. He didn't want toast or cereal or porridge or sandwiches or apple shortcake or chocolate brownies or lemon cake or ginger crunch. Dear child.

I delivered him and Ellie to the bus stop, noticing in passing that he wasn't wearing shoes. Oh well, there was only a light frost this morning. Then I continued up the road to Val's to borrow enough milk for afternoon smoko.

I rushed home again to get my scones out of the oven. They should have been puffy and luscious and golden brown; they were pale and flabby and uninteresting. That's what happens when you forget the baking powder.

So I danced in rage for a little while, gave the shearers the lemon cake meant for afternoon smoko and spent some time trying to think of something to bake that contained neither butter nor milk. Couldn't do it – all I could come up with was lemon cake, which is made with oil, and I couldn't give them two lemon cakes in one day. Grandma once told me that when she was newly married and hadn't yet learnt to cook, she fed the shearers on ginger and apple muffins for three weeks straight, because it was the only recipe she'd mastered. But at the time Grandma was twenty-one years old and completely adorable. Being considerably older and much less adorable than my sainted grandmother, I went back to Val's place for butter, and made Afghan biscuits. And then discovered, on icing them, that we were out of icing sugar …

James and the shearers drank that box of beer at the end of the day.

Just. Saying.

Saturday 23 May

Now that we're out of lockdown, the repair man has come to look at our fridge and pronounced it irrevocably dead. And we can't buy a new one the same size because they don't make them anymore. Not a single fridge on the market will fit into the fridge-sized gap in our kitchen. We asked Val if we could keep the one we borrowed during lockdown and buy her a new one, and she said of course we could keep it but we couldn't possibly pay her. She doesn't need the fridge, it was in the way in any case, and why can't we just graciously accept it as a gift? So we thanked her very much and put the money for a new fridge into her account. Because we're not the sort of people who take fridges without paying for them. Or, to pick another example *entirely* at random, pay a box of beer for a sheep and then help drink the beer. (Goodness, I really do need to let that go.)

Now that Val's fridge is staying, I spent an hour this morning removing its door and putting it on the other way so we could open it without it hitting the wall. Ellie helped me hold the door up and Blake provided suggestions and advice. I broke one piece of plastic and had two screws left over when I was finished, which I felt was overall a good effort. (Like in *To Kill a Mockingbird*, where Jem made a wonderful job of reassembling his watch with only three bits left over, but it still wouldn't go.)

On being asked how you get rid of old fridges if you don't want to throw them down a bank into the bush (the recycling centre in town won't take them), James suggested we keep it and turn it into a garden feature. We could tip it on its back and fill it with ice and beer when visitors come. He knows someone who makes swans out of old tyres, and he'll get me a couple to go with it. Dear James. So caring and thoughtful.

Amy and I went out for lunch in town today, leaving our families at home. It was *lovely*. After our meal we had a look around the shops, just to round out a delightful expedition. Amy bought a jersey and I bought a pair of jeans. Then we paused in front of an antique shop whose owner was sitting outside the door. She had a clipboard on a little table beside her for contact tracing of customers, but she explained to us that she couldn't let us in; she wasn't well enough. Unless we wanted to look at furniture, which she would haul into the doorway to show us. All very perplexing. I wonder why she feels that sitting on the pavement is an acceptable health risk, but letting people into the shop is not? Actually, I wonder why she bothered to open – if opening you could call it – at all?

Ellie asked this evening if the woolshed floor is made of concrete or marble. Bless. Marble, of course, to go with the mahogany wool board.

Sunday 24 May

Blake had a friend over today, a very nice little girl from his class at school. They decided to be friends last summer holidays, but they carefully ignore one another at school so as to avoid being teased. In honour of her visit, Blake tidied his room, unasked. The two of them came with me to feed the palm kernel. They ran down the hills and crept up on sheep to scare them and fought duels with flannel-leaf-stem staffs, and were generally cute and wholesome and athletic.

After lunch they went on an expedition to climb the big chestnut tree. They walked home up the road, and staggered in with a big armful of rubbish each. They had combed the roadsides and picked up every beer bottle and scrap of silage wrap between Dan's driveway and ours.

This girl is obviously a brilliant influence on my erratic son. I hope they get married when they grow up.

Monday 25 May

I had a phone call at lunchtime from the manager of the Kiwi House – the nice Indian man from the liquor shop at the north end of town had just rung to say he had a baby kingfisher in a box. The local bird rescue lady is on holiday, and Ellie adores rearing baby birds – would I like to take it? Sure. So I went down to the liquor shop at the north end of town, where the following dialogue ensued.

> *Me: Hi! I've come to get the kingfisher.*
> *Him: Very good. We have Kingfisher. You want twelve or twenty-four?*
> *Me: No, no – I mean the little bird. The baby bird.*
> *Him (extremely puzzled): But we no stock birds. We have Kingfisher beer.*
> *Me: Oh, I'm sorry; I was told you had a baby kingfisher …*

His English is a bit shaky, and the more I explained the more confused he got, and I started to get the impression he was wondering if I was crazy, so I slunk out and went to the liquor shop at the *south* end of town. And there, on a freezing cold windowsill, sitting on a bar towel, was an adult kingfisher that had obviously flown into a window and concussed itself. The man behind the counter held out his hand for it to hop onto a finger, at which it panicked and ricocheted around the window frame in a way that couldn't have done its headache any good at all. I wrapped it in the bar towel and took it back to work, gave it a drink of water out of a syringe and some pain relief, and put it in a box in the hot-water cupboard.

Tuesday 26 May

This morning the kingfisher was bright-eyed, bushy-tailed and absolutely furious. I opened up its box outside behind the clinic, and it clattered its beak, gave me a filthy look, jumped up onto the side of the box, decided not, after all, to waste the time and energy required to stab me in the eye, and headed like an arrow for the river. Excellent.

Today Sophie and I vasectomised fifteen little bulls, with another ten to go tomorrow. Last year it was an appalling job; this year the bulls were four months younger and 100 kilograms lighter, I had all the equipment nicely organised, and we had a delightful morning. We ran them up the race in groups of five, vaccinated, sedated, blood-tested and gave them all penicillin, and then vasectomised them one at a time in the head bail. The only thing I didn't get right was the sedation. The first ten went like clockwork, but by the time we loaded up the third race-full, they'd been standing in the yards for two hours and were so relaxed – or maybe so bored – that the same dose of sedative put them right to sleep, and we had to prod each one to its feet and shout continuously in its ear to keep it standing. Human surgeons miss a lot, I think. How often do they end up feverishly clamping sections of vas deferens while their patient sags and sways and then crumples gently into the mud puddle in the bottom of the race? There must be so much less excitement in operating under controlled, sterile conditions.

Wednesday 27 May

The palm kernel is finished! Hooray!

This frees up the old tractor, which can now be used for spraying gorse – my next job. I'm not particularly excited about this, but on the bright side, walking up and down hills dragging a spray hose should do wonders for the firmness of my thighs.

Today, as on every business day for the last five weeks, the tights we ordered online for Ellie failed to arrive. She is getting very bitter about it, especially since Blake's new spinning reel, which was ordered a fortnight later, came last Friday.

Thursday 28 May

After dropping the kids at the bus, I carried on down the farm to plant some trees in a very nice corner of wetland that will be all the nicer with a little grove of kahikatea trees in it. A noble and praiseworthy exercise, but next time I dig holes in a swamp I think I'll wait until the frost melts. My fingers got colder and colder, and the rest of me got hotter and hotter, so that by the time I'd finished my hands were like ice blocks and my glasses had fogged up with steam.

After de-icing and de-fogging, James and I went to the dentist. Several hours and $500 later (and that's before he gets two fillings and they pull out two of my wisdom teeth – here come the good times) we were home again, having a coffee before going down the farm.

I wandered into our room and found James turning a polar fleece jersey around in his hands. 'I'm just looking for the food stains to figure out where the front is,' he explained.

Well, I knew what I was getting myself into. It's not like he used to be any classier. On our first Valentine's Day together he gave me a card with a cartoon dog on the front and a poem inside:

> *Roses are red, violets are blue,*
> *Sometimes I drink from the toilet.*
> *The end.*

Friday 29 May

I spent a happy morning refilling my new line of bait stations along the river at the back of the farm. Half the line follows a nice dry stretch of riverbank through the bush – lovely bush, all full of fat pungas with mossy trunks – and the other half skirts a swamp. Every bait station on the dry half of the line was empty, and every one alongside the swamp was full. Evidently rats don't like getting their feet wet any more than I do. I'll have to move the line.

Still no tights. Ellie is very disappointed. On learning this afternoon that, yet again, they hadn't come, she said bitterly, 'I'll be in my room. Probably for the rest of my life.' Which seems a little drastic, considering that she's appropriated my yoga pants and two pairs of leggings to fill her current wardrobe deficit.

Winter

Reasons that winter is awesome:

- *It's the proper weather for flannelette pyjamas. And flannelette pyjamas are my favourite clothes in all the world. (Equal with the onesie, that glorious fusion of practicality and style.)*
- *It's totally morally acceptable to put on pyjamas as soon as it gets dark. It gets dark at five. That's fourteen happy pyjama-clad hours out of twenty-four.*
- *Soup. Stew. Gravy. All so delicious and warm and satisfying.*
- *Calving cows. Absolutely the most satisfying veterinary job. You turn up, you diagnose the problem, and you fix it. (Mostly.)*
- *Winter sports. (That's a lie. I resent spending Saturday mornings standing on the edge of a rugby field watching my child get trampled into the mud. But I realise I should enjoy it. Everyone else seems to.)*

Monday 1 June

We've had an action-packed Queen's Birthday weekend. Mum and Dad have been here, we've been on an expedition to see the tallest tree in New Zealand (the start of the walk is only 40 minutes' drive away; who knew?) and had friends over for tea. Mum and I visited her favourite shoe shop, where she bought a gorgeous pair of bright orange sneakers which I plan to steal as soon as possible, and Dad fixed the kitchen cabinets so they all open and close with smooth clicking sounds rather than grating and shuddering and needing to be hit in exactly the right place. James and I do not excel at home maintenance – we both tend towards the approach of kicking things to see if that fixes them.

Tuesday 2 June

The tights arrived! And so did a letter offering Ellie a place in the hostel for next year. We're so pleased she's got in – and so sorry to be sending her away.

James made dinner tonight. He fried onion, carrot and ginger, and then added udon noodles, soya sauce and beaten egg. He served this bizarre combination on focaccia. I do wish he didn't think that recipes are beneath him.

Wednesday 3 June

Sean and Amy's smallest girl started school today. She has a rainbow unicorn backpack (pink, with pompoms) that's nearly as big as she is, a rainbow unicorn lunchbox and a rainbow unicorn pencil case. For years she's been wistfully watching the others climb onto the bus, and today she got to do it too. She nearly burst with pride and excitement. It was incredibly cute.

I learnt a little about Sophie's love life today, as we spayed cats. And it confirmed that I am repressed, inhibited and embarrassingly out of date. Out of date or not, I'm *appalled* to learn that sending pictures of your bits via Snapchat is not only an accepted but an expected part of dating these days. *Why*? Is it supposed to be arousing? Or is it part of a standard checklist? (Do you have a penis? Ah, yes, there it is. No scabs or discharges? Very well, then, let's meet for coffee.) The potential for shame and humiliation, if you're sending these pictures to people you barely know, seems so high. Although not, I suppose, quite as high as the level of shame and humiliation that would come from hitting the wrong button and sending them to people you know well …

Apparently, kids' rugby *will* go ahead this year after all, starting next term. Which will make the end of season later than usual, so that it will coincide neatly with lambing and calving. Blake is thrilled. His parents are not.

Thursday 4 June

It was raining this morning, so that although James has taken the front-end loader off the old tractor and put the spray unit on, I couldn't spray gorse. I was, of course, crushed. I am going to stay in my pyjamas all day instead, and write. It will be *amazing*.

Friday 5 June

Yesterday's amazing writing day was less productive than I had planned. I went to sleep on the couch, woke up, reread what I've already written, didn't like it much, read a book instead and went back to sleep. Which is a poor effort, really, from someone who claims she wants to be a writer. I did, however, make osso bucco and peanut butter chocolate chip biscuits, both of which were delicious.

Once again, it's too wet to spray today, and I just spent a very happy hour planting succulents in the gaps in the stone ha-ha at the bottom of the lawn. Gardening in the rain is a very underrated activity. But my happiness is fading fast beneath the cold and menacing shadow of this afternoon's wisdom tooth extractions. And we're picking up Ellie's best friend on the way home, and I'm on call this weekend. Although Sophie, bless her, has offered to cover any calls tonight. Still, I think I might have bitten off more than I can chew. Especially with two less teeth ...

7.30 p.m.

The dental appointment seemed, at first, to be going beautifully. I didn't even feel the anaesthetic injections, the dentist and the dental nurse were pleasant and smiley, there was good music on the radio ...

After tugging at tooth one for a while, the dentist said there wasn't very much room, so he'd just switch to tooth two. Once it was out, he'd be able to manoeuvre his forceps properly.

Tooth two slid out like a dream. Back to tooth one.

Tooth one was going nowhere. Would the nurse just pop out and tell James we wouldn't be long (he had the next appointment)? Meanwhile, the dentist would split my uncooperative tooth in half for easier manipulation.

He split the tooth in half with a drill and started levering it out.

The crown broke off the tooth, leaving the roots behind.

The dentist closed his eyes for a second, then explained he'd have to cut a gum flap and get at the broken roots from the side. A bit of a shame, because it would take a little longer to heal, but not a problem.

He cut the gum flap.

He burred and picked and levered.

He asked the nurse to tell James he'd have to come back for his appointment another day.

He took another X-ray.

He consulted with a colleague.

He levered a little more.

He explained, with a fine sheen of sweat upon his brow, that he couldn't get the root out, so he'd have to try to destroy the nerve, sew the flap shut, send me home on antibiotics and painkillers, and get me an appointment with an oral surgeon.

The poor man. I know exactly how he felt – that mixture of shame, disbelief and self-reproach that comes from starting a perfectly straightforward procedure and having every possible thing go wrong. It was a 45-minute appointment, and I was in there for two and a half hours.

I'm feeling fine. I've had two types of painkiller to replace the local anaesthetic, and my mouth isn't bothering me at all. I hope it's not still bothering the poor dentist!

Sunday 7 June

On-call weekend and tooth roots both very manageable so far. I took Blake with me to the clinic on Saturday morning, so he didn't sit at home brooding about Ellie having a friend to stay while he was alone. There was not a single call and barely a single customer, but he had a wonderful time talking to Jess and playing with the coffee machine and the office chairs. As we pulled out of the car park at twelve to go home again the phone rang – a down cow for a farmer who belonged, until the first of June, to the furthest distant branch of the practice. He has now moved further north, well out of the area we cover, but has yet to sign up with a new vet clinic. I bought us some sushi for lunch, and we drove for an hour and a half to look at the cow. She had done the splits on the yard and was sitting in a paddock with her legs out, frog-style. She had no sensation at all in either foot when I jabbed them with a needle. Diagnosis: serious injury to the roots of the femoral nerves, with recovery time of about a month, during which she would have to be bedded down on something soft, lifted twice a day, and prevented from crawling and making it worse. Poor prognosis, and logistics of nursing almost impossible. Advised shooting her, and drove an hour and a half home.

*

The next call, at 4 p.m., was to a seizuring heifer. I made it two kilometres down the road before they called back to say she'd died.

On Sunday morning I saw a sick cow. High fever, dull and weak and generally miserable, with foul-smelling diarrhoea. Probably salmonella. Gave her antibiotics and pain relief and vitamin B1 and ketol, which should make her feel much better about life.

On Sunday afternoon I pulled a teeny-weeny calf out of a heifer. It was as big as a Jack Russell, and it lay on the yard and yelled at the top of its voice. Its mother was terrified of it, and when we let her out, she fled to the furthest corner of the yard and stood watching it in horror. The farmer asked me to put it down, and I very nearly asked him if I could take it home for Ellie – but sanity prevailed. Breathing through undercooked lungs is a massive struggle, and the poor little thing would almost certainly have died overnight, if not before. I put it down.

Tuesday 9 June

We had an Incident at work this morning. I spayed a cat – a smooth, routine procedure – and Emma carried her away to recover. She woke up, Emma extubated her ... and as she pulled the endotracheal tube out, the cat bit it cleanly in half and sucked the end back down into her trachea.

Instant panic. We tried to pull the tube out with a pair of forceps, the cat fought and coughed and spluttered, the tube vanished completely.

We anaesthetised her again. I blew two veins in the process – not *entirely* my fault; she had veins like tissue paper.

We couldn't see or reach the tube. Sophie came in, and we both rang small-animal vets in other branches of the practice for advice. One told us to swing her around upside down and pray to the gods of gravity, and the other told us we'd have to do a tracheotomy. We swung her like the spin cycle on a washing machine, which really isn't ideal for a patient who just had abdominal surgery. The tube stayed snugly at the thoracic inlet, where the neck joins the rib cage. We could palpate its end, and that was it.

I tried desperately to massage the tube up the trachea, with the poor cat hanging upside down. Nope.

We topped up the anaesthetic, thus blowing all the remaining available veins, and started a tracheotomy. By now there were four vets in the room, and then Bill dropped in for a cup of tea, so we dragged him in as consultant surgeon.

I cut down between the jugular vein and the carotid artery and the vagus nerve and other spine-chillingly important structures, and eventually got to the trachea. I made a little hole in it, poked the forceps in, and pulled out ten centimetres of plastic ET tube. I've never been so pleased to see a bit of plastic in my entire life.

That cat is a *heroine*. An hour after her near-death experience, she was sitting up and purring. By five she looked as bright as a button, and when I went back into the clinic at seven to see a sick little dog she meowed insistently until I took her out and cuddled her.

For dinner tonight, James the culinary artiste made pasta with broccoli, onion and carrot, all covered in white sauce. He was wounded by the kids' lack of enthusiasm for this taste sensation, so I stretched the truth and said it was delicious. He then explained proudly that he never quite knows what dinner will be until it's ready. Yes, we'd noticed. (In the interests of justice, I should say that last night he produced a perfectly respectable, barely peculiar meal of sausages, potato cakes and fried slices of fresh pineapple.)

Wednesday 10 June

Today I visited a mob of ewes to investigate a mysterious ill-thrift and death problem – young ewes that begin to lose weight, develop diarrhoea and eventually die. The farmer gave them all a vitamin B12 injection a few weeks ago, but it didn't really help.

When were they last drenched? I asked.

Never. He's breeding a line of tough, worm-resistant sheep.

He's almost positive the problem is a trace element deficiency.

I'm almost positive the problem is worms. If it looks like a duck, and quacks like a duck, chances are it's going to be a duck.

I've taken some blood and faecal samples, so we shall see.

My broken-off tooth roots are beginning to make their presence felt. I have an emergency appointment with the oral surgeon next Tuesday (it's a workday, and there's a lot of work booked in, but the next available appointment was the end of July and I'm just not selfless enough to wait that long). I wonder how my mouth will be feeling by then? Thank goodness for Voltaren and codeine.

Thursday 11 June

I have an email from the CEO at work saying that, for the first time in my life, I've brought in sufficient fees to earn a bonus for the December to March quarter. It's $900, before tax. Awesome!

I also have an email from the oral surgeon's office, estimating my tooth root extraction at $1800. This makes me feel better about charging $300 to see a dog after hours on Monday and put it on a drip, which seemed criminally expensive. It also spares me the agony of deciding how to spend my bonus.

Friday 12 June

Spent the day teat-sealing heifers. Although we're now at level-one restrictions, meaning the technicians can work again, one has broken her finger, one has broken her arm and one is busy leaving her husband. We did 110 in the morning and 140 in the afternoon. Although they were nice, friendly little heifers – the odd one tried to leap forwards into the feed bins or backwards into the pit, but none of them were the kick-you-to-death-as-soon-as-look-at-you variety – it was still a long, hard day.

I called our medical insurance hotline, just on the off-chance that they might cover tooth root removals, and they do! Not only that, but both James and I have earned a hundred-dollar voucher because we haven't claimed anything for years. Ordered myself a gorgeous merino hoodie costing $240 off the internet on the strength of it, and now feel slightly queasy with guilt.

Saturday 13 June

Ellie has lined the bath with pillows and retired there with a book. It looks beautifully comfortable.

We went to Hobbiton today – it's only the middle of the month, and James has spent *four days* off farm already! (Part days, and two of them were tooth-related, but still.) We were only moderately enthusiastic about going to Hobbiton, but Blake has been dying to visit the place for years. The last ten kilometres of road there were very windy, and the first thing he did on arrival was to throw up in the car park.

After that inauspicious start, we had a great time. Our tour guide was lovely and the set is beautiful. All the little gardens around the hobbit holes are landscaped with plants I wish I had in my garden. Blake and the guide quoted lines from the movies to each other and debated whether Elijah Wood was a good casting choice for Frodo (they felt, on balance, that he was a bit of a drip). We had a complimentary drink at the Green Dragon pub and then an enormous pizza lunch at the cafe, and bought Blake a framed map of Middle Earth. 'Mum,' he hissed as we were leaving, 'I'm having a *blast*.'

James zipped his cell phone into the pocket of his good sweatshirt and then the zip stuck. He got it out, on reaching home, by cutting not one but two holes through the side of the sweatshirt with a pair of scissors (he missed the pocket with his first hole). When asked why he hadn't cut the pocket on the *inside* rather than savaging his best hoodie he looked sheepish but responded by tossing his head and saying, 'Didn't want to.'

Words fail me.

Sunday 14 June

Something, James informs me, Must Be Done about the pigs. They've dug up about a third of their paddock.

As previously, I have earnestly agreed with him.

I know perfectly well that when he says Something Must Be Done, he actually means You Fix It. Having spent half an hour last night sewing up the holes in his sweatshirt, I feel disinclined to oblige him.

This morning Blake and I took the ute on an expedition to my favourite nursery to buy native trees to plant by the creek. I snuck in a selection of nice flowering shrubs. A viburnum, a grape, a flowering quince, a really lovely silver-veined Virginia creeper … I'm dying to get them all planted, but between helping James dag lambs to go to the works and taking Ellie into town for her netball muster, I ran out of daylight.

The lambs weren't all finished by dinnertime – I went back to the woolshed with James and helped him from seven till eight, and then he finished up and got home by nine. A nice, relaxing way to spend a Sunday evening.

Monday 15 June

Today was my ideal workday. I visited my very favourite farmers and vaccinated their herd, went to a sheep milking farm to post-mortem a dead ewe, scanned some heifers, vaccinated an adorable rabbit, looked at an even more adorable puppy with a sprained hock, saw a kiwi with a mouth infection and a farm dog with a ruptured gastrocnemius muscle. I *love* mixed practice.

The lab results from last week's dying sheep case show that many – although not all – of the faecal samples contain a significant number of worm eggs. And there are significantly more worm eggs in the thin group than in the fat group. I have reported this to the farmer, who politely disagrees with my conclusion that worms are the primary issue. The worms, he says, are probably secondary to a trace element deficiency.

Oh well, it's his money. I've requested a full range of trace element tests. I'm going to feel really stupid if he's right and I'm wrong …

While cruising the supermarket aisles, I spotted a big roll of dog poo collection bags. I was very excited. They'll be *perfect* bait bags (bait stays crisp and dry and delicious to rats for much longer if you wrap it in a plastic bag) and I'm chronically short of bags in this post-single-use-plastic-bag era, even though Val and Amy and Melissa all save bread bags for me when they remember. On reading the label on my new bags, I discovered that while they aren't biodegradable, they *are* recyclable. Who, I wonder, washes out and recycles a bag they've used for collecting dog shit?

I'm getting my tooth roots dug out tomorrow. Thank goodness. I'm very grateful for the large amounts of painkillers the dentist prescribed, but I've been living on them for ten days now, and I'm starting to worry about my stomach lining.

Tuesday 16 June, 5 p.m.

Val, bless her, drove me to the oral surgeon this morning. I remember nothing after: 'This is midazolam, it will take about thirty seconds to kick in ...' But I assume my tooth roots are all gone, because I feel like I've been kicked in the jaw by a horse.

Sophie just sent a text message to say she'd do my on-call for me. I hadn't even thought about organising a swap. Sophie is wonderful.

Going back to bed. Perhaps for the rest of the week.

Wednesday 17 June

The sheep scanner, an excellent chap and a wonderful source of interesting gossip about the neighbours, came this morning. He scans flat out; James and Thomas pen up and push ewes into the crate; I mark singles, triplets, lates and empties with spray paint and draft off thin ewes and empties. We've done it like that for the last ten years, and everyone is extremely efficient except me. I am only moderately efficient; occasionally I lose focus and stand idly with paint can in hand while the scanner says gently, 'Late. Late. *Late*.'

But since today I qualified as walking wounded, everyone was obliged to be impressed by my nobility and devotion to duty rather than irritated by my incompetence. I was impressed myself by the time we finished, and took my aching jaw straight home to bed.

The results were wonderful – 179 percent (179 lambs seen per hundred ewes), and only 77 ewes having triplets. Two years ago, when we *didn't* have a horrible drought over mating, we had more than 200 triplet-bearing ewes. Triplets are no fun at all –

the ewes are far more likely to die over lambing, and their lambs are far more likely to die afterwards – so it's wonderful to be expecting so few of them. A nice silver lining to the drought.

Thursday 18 June

This morning I felt great, and went down the farm to plant twenty-five trees and put in three new bait stations. After which, like yesterday, I felt considerably less great, and came back home to bed.

Amy's smallest girl got off the bus this afternoon in a pair of school tracksuit bottoms. On being questioned by her mother, she explained, 'I just keep forgetting not to wet my pants.' She's not embarrassed at all; it's just one of those things. I'm so impressed – one of my worst memories is wetting my knickers at the top of the school jungle gym, aged five. I was distraught, and thought I could never hold up my head in public again. Little Emily's approach is so much more sensible.

The trace element testing results for last week's mysterious dying sheep are in. All normal. Ha!

9 p.m.

James just got home from a board of trustees meeting at the school, and told me in awed tones that when Wendy had *her* wisdom teeth out, they had to chisel the roots out of the bone. Poor Wendy, he said. It must have been horrific.

Um, yes, I said, radiating courage and nobility, that's what the surgeon did with mine on Tuesday.

Friday 19 June

It was raining today, and I was looking forward to staying inside and writing. My princess is currently trying to break her erstwhile kidnappers out of a burning building, and naturally I'm keen to find out how it goes.

Before settling down to write, I vacuumed, folded a mountain of washing, cleaned the kitchen, paid the bills, reconciled last month's accounts, collated the last quarter's farm fuel invoices, paid the GST and filled in an online claim for my dental surgery. Which all took till lunchtime, and my concentration is at its very lowest ebb in the early afternoon. Bugger. But I could never have concentrated on the princess and her adventures with all those other jobs looming over me.

Somehow, after swearing we wouldn't let it happen, we have accumulated four after-school activities a week again. Tuesday is Blake's rugby practice, Wednesday is Ellie's dancing, Thursday she has netball practice and Blake has a *second* rugby practice (not at the same time, so that will be two hours spent kicking around in town), and Friday is Ellie's netball game. Blake's rugby games are on Saturday mornings. It's ridiculous.

On the bright side, what with the current border quarantine debacles (most notably the two Covid-positive English ladies who were released early from quarantine, untested, and who drove the length of the North Island before feeling unwell and getting themselves diagnosed), the country might soon be back in lockdown.

Monday 22 June

While pregnancy-testing a mob of beef cows today, we drafted an empty heifer into the pen where I was standing. She turned out to be the panic-when-separated-from-the-mob kind of heifer, and decided that she'd have to kill both me and the farmer if she were to have any chance of surviving herself.

The farmer shut her into a separate little pen with railings too high (probably) to jump, showing exceptional bravery and using himself as bait to lure her in. With markedly less bravery, I stood and watched from two pens away, poised for further flight if required. For the rest of the time I was there she watched me through the rails with fixed, unblinking hatred, occasionally pawing the ground with a front hoof. It was very off-putting.

Both kids had colds this morning and spent the day at home, tolerance for runny noses at school being currently very low. When James got home for lunch, he found them frantically cleaning their bedrooms, with all the furniture piled in the hall. Definitely the sort of behaviour to be encouraged.

Wednesday 24 June

I woke up this morning with the kids' cold, and decided to go to work anyway. I have since been reflecting on the wisdom of this decision, and the comparative inconveniences caused by me calling in sick on a busy workday versus me wandering around the community potentially spreading coronavirus. I don't think for a moment that I have coronavirus, but that's not the point. Poor form. Will do better in future.

Quite apart from potential disease transmission, I was far from my best today. I automatically turned left out of the car park behind the clinic when I should have turned right, corrected at the corner and then turned left *again* at the next intersection. I did eventually manage to head north rather than south, only to reach my destination without the parcel I was supposed to be dropping off to a farmer. Then I failed to find any reason for a heifer's raging temperature on physical examination and poked my needle right through the scruff of a cat's neck, thus wasting the vaccine I had brought out for it. Usually I bring extra vaccine in case of such accidents, but not today.

The sole bright spot was watching two small children playing in the mud beside the cattle yards. It was cold and drizzling, but they were totally happy. The little girl was wearing her favourite pink sparkly tutu over her wet-weather gear. Their mother, who was loading cows up the race with great efficiency and skill, said that they're entirely fearless and she's had to tell them that if they go in the paddock with her horse it will kick their heads off and they'll die. She feels a bit guilty about trying to scare them, but figures it's better than having them stood on by a horse.

Blake and I started reading Terry Pratchett's *Nation* tonight. He asked many searching questions about whether the hero and heroine get married at the end, and expressed great dissatisfaction when I admitted that they don't. Blake, like me, wants to make sure a story's going to end happily before he invests in it. I promised him it would be okay, but he remains sceptical.

Thursday 25 June

Resolved to be a more responsible citizen today, I called the dentist, where I'm supposed to be going for a check-up this morning, to tell them I've got a cold.

'Oh,' said the very nice receptionist. 'We *would* really like to see you ... Do you think it's just the common cold?'

'I think so,' I said.

'So just a cold? No runny nose or sore throat?'

I admitted I had both a runny nose and a sore throat, and we decided it would be better not to come in. What sort of cold *doesn't* come standard with a runny nose and a sore throat, I wonder?

Friday 26 June

Spent the morning walking around in circles in the bush, trying to find the bait station line that was shown to me a few months ago. Pleasant, but frustrating – last time I was there I wrote myself a number of notes on my phone, such as: *After 102 turn hard left to 103, dead end, then back across face to J loop.* Today I found 103 randomly at the bottom of a ridge, couldn't find any sign of 102, and plunged onwards across the creek onto an entirely different line, missing the rest of J loop entirely. Never mind; I found at least twenty bait stations, almost all of them empty. Now they are full. More rats will die. More birds will live.

After lunch I went down to school assembly, where Blake and Ellie both received badges.

It was pyjama day, and the school library was filled with children and staff wearing monster dressing-gowns, unicorn onesies and hamburger slippers. They looked fabulous.

Saturday 27 June

Ellie came with me to Saturday morning clinic today, and we'd barely settled down with hot drinks when we had a call to one dead cow, one bloated cow, one down in the race and one frothing at the mouth.

It turned out that the worker let the dry cows onto the feed pad to finish up the last of the maize left behind by the milking cows – there wasn't much maize left, only a mouthful each – but instead of putting the whole mob on at once he let them trickle in and help themselves. Which means, I suspect, that the first ten cows helped themselves to ten kilos of maize each and nobody else got any. The problem with piling ten kilos of maize into a rumen as a one-off is that the right bacteria to digest it aren't there, so it ferments and turns to acid, poisoning the cow and burning holes in the lining of her rumen. It must be horrendously painful.

I filled up the three down cows with calcium and pain relief and penicillin and drenched them with magnesium slurry (like Quik-Eze for cows), and we pulled one that kept trying to lie down in the electric fence out into the middle of the paddock. There were another half-dozen standing sadly in a corner, so I left the worker more supplies to treat those ones too, once he'd walked them to the shed. I expect at least the worst two will die – it's a horrible thing to have happened.

Sunday 28 June

Bean the cat has taken to waking us in the morning by clawing her way up the side of the mattress onto James's side of the bed, standing on his head, continuing across us both to the very edge of my side and swiping my glasses off my bedside table onto the floor. Her eyesight is pretty poor now, and sometimes it takes her quite a while to find the glasses, but she manages it eventually.

This morning she roused me from a dream in which I had been carefully splitting my dead manager's head open with a sharp shovel to let the formalin in and better preserve his brain, but then he opened his eyes. So I rushed him to hospital, driving on the wrong side of the road down many curvy tunnels filled with oncoming traffic, stopping to buy a ticket for the toll road from a building decorated like the reception of a movie theatre, full of random passages and staircases, and with no signage. Now I'll never know whether we made it.

I just rang yesterday's farmer to see how the acidosis cows went. Most of the ones we treated got up, but four of the ones that were still on their feet and that he treated after I'd gone have died, although he gave them all the drugs I left him.

It makes no sense. Those ones weren't as sick as the ones I treated. The only difference between the two groups is that I gave my ones injectable calcium, using up all I had in the ute, so I left him oral calcium for the rest. Maybe calcium isn't absorbed very well from a damaged rumen, and they died of milk fever. Shit, shit, shit. I wish I'd gone and got him a box of injectable calcium. And I wish he'd rung me yesterday when they started dying.

9 p.m.
A nice, peaceful day on call. I spent an hour this morning operating on a cow with a displaced stomach – the whole thing went beautifully, like a textbook, which makes a pleasant

change. Then this afternoon I tried to make a dog who'd eaten rat bait throw it up again. He had a stomach of cast iron, that dog. Eventually he spat up a pathetic little bit of froth, so I sent him away with ten days' worth of vitamin K to counteract the bait he'd absorbed.

I made a recipe a friend gave me for dinner – hearty chicken and vegetable soup. It was so hearty that it was really more of a chicken and vegetable slurry, but it was great. And slopping it into bowls like prison food provided the children some amusement, which was nice, because they didn't have the most exciting weekend.

Monday 29 June

I've received a Facebook message from a very nice woman who writes that she particularly enjoys my books because they're so easy to read that she flies through them even though she's dyslexic. I am resolving to take this as a compliment.

Tuesday 30 June

I spent from eight thirty to eleven this morning standing on a box, vaccinating 400 cows as they came around on a very old, very slow rotary platform. Enjoyed it thoroughly – it reminded me of a colleague who once said that he couldn't understand why vets all want to rush off and be consultants and specialists. That's *hard*. Mundane, routine jobs are easy, and have the added advantage of leaving most of your brain free for thinking about sex. (Not that I spent two and a half hours standing on a box and thinking about sex. Honest.)

The rest of the day was filled with stocktaking. Last stocktake, we were out by many thousands of dollars, and our manager is very keen not to repeat the debacle. He had a stressful day, with much pacing and checking of barcodes. The rest of us enjoyed the change of routine, especially the pizza for lunch and the rainbow unicorn cupcakes, chips and beer for after work. Life is so much more comfortable when you're a carefree and irresponsible underling.

Wednesday 1 July

James spent the morning knocking down the old, broken sheep yards at the back of the farm, ready to put up new ones. And he discovered that the yards are paved with bricks. Beautiful old red-clay bricks, the type that landscapers sell for three dollars apiece. Whoopee!

Thursday 2 July

Too tired to sleep. This is due to spending the morning scraping the grass and blackberry off my 500 beautiful new bricks, digging them up, stacking them on a pallet (James helped, and loaded the pallet on the back of the ute with the tractor), and then unloading them at home onto another pallet by myself.

In the afternoon I bagged ten kilos of bait and walked around a large, steep block of bush, refilling bait stations. It took me three hours.

After all that saintliness, I lapsed badly at dinnertime by deciding that although my family had thanked me for their meals, they hadn't thanked me nicely enough, and I shouted at them, reducing Ellie to tears. Not cool.

Friday 3 July

We had the most beautiful frost this morning, and the air was sharp and crisp and tangy. Just before sunrise about 10,000 starlings, who have taken to roosting in the bamboo hedge at the woolshed (it now smells like a chicken farm), came swirling across the sky like leaves in a gale. Gorgeous.

After breakfast, Thomas came to talk to James about helping him lay out a water pipe. He wouldn't come in, so they stood on either side of the open door for twenty minutes, while all the warm air in the kitchen and living room escaped, and grunted at one another. James and Thomas conduct whole long, complex conversations in grunts – it's quite fascinating. I suspect they're actually telepathic, but they don't realise it. Surely it's impossible to communicate that you'll meet at nine thirty tomorrow at the bottom yards in grunts alone.

Ellie's netball game this evening was most exciting. For one thing, her team actually got some goals (they still lost 32–7, but it was an improvement on last week). Their shooter was amazing. He was only about four feet tall, but he normally plays basketball, and he shot goals, apparently without even looking at the hoop, from all over the circle. The other bit of excitement was that the lights, which are very old and prone to overheating, went out halfway through the game. The kids could barely see one another, let alone tell who was on whose team. Eventually someone had the brilliant idea of parking their car pointing at the court and leaving the lights on.

Saturday 4 July

Last night it occurred to us that the school holidays had begun and we had, as usual, made no plans whatsoever for fun family outings. The bright idea that we could spend a couple of nights in Taupo ended in the discovery that everyone else in the country had apparently had the same idea and booked all the affordable accommodation.

Still, we've made a good start to the holidays. Blake and Ellie and I spent the afternoon luxuriating at the newly opened local day spa. (James spent it digging in Thomas's new pipe. Sucks to be him.) Mum had given me a voucher for a float in one of the spa's new Dreampods for my birthday, and I booked the kids in for half an hour's massage each while I floated.

It was so cool. The floatation pod is shaped like a big egg. You shower and get in, pulling the top down after you, and bob in the salty water, watching soft lights play over the egg's roof. I floated for a few minutes and then thought, 'Very relaxing, but could potentially get a little bit boring ...' Then I thought, 'Someone's snoring,' followed closely by, 'Oh. Me.' And about three seconds later the time-to-get-out music started.

I showered the salt off, rubbed on a selection of gorgeous creams, and wafted out, to be greeted by two delighted children who say that no matter how good floating was, it couldn't *possibly* have been as nice as their massages. They had soft lavender pads over their eyes and warm towels on their backs, and the masseuse had the smoothest, gentlest hands you could possibly imagine. She even did Ellie's hair in a beautiful, intricate French plait.

I think we could quite easily become accustomed to a life of luxury.

Sunday 5 July

Blake and I spent a happy hour laying out bricks this morning, moving them around until we achieved a graceful curve. It looks really good. In preparation for constructing my path, I then watched a step-by-step explanatory video on YouTube. It was a depressingly professional-looking video, involving levels and concrete and special patented plastic edging. Who can be bothered with that sort of carry-on? Surely it'll look fine if I just dig a trench in the lawn, line it with crusher dust and tuck the bricks into it, level with the ground? Checking Google for an inspirational quote confirming this approach, I've found one by Voltaire: *The best is the enemy of the good.* That's right. Better a good-enough path that gets built than an absolutely perfect path that doesn't because I'm too intimidated by the thought of all that concrete to start.

Monday 6 July

Today, so as to add a spice of excitement to a routine blood-testing job, I took a tray of 100 blood tubes out to sample 99 bulls. Optimistic, when you can expect to blow at least one in ten tubes. I managed to scratch up another handful out of the back of my ute, and then I and the vet student who came with me blood-tested with grim concentration and crossed fingers. Luckily, she was a particularly capable and efficient vet student. We finished with two tubes to spare. Whew.

Tuesday 7 July

Very stressful morning. A lovely girl who's studying to be a veterinary technician brought in her fearful, aggressive dog to spay, and asked if she could stay and watch the surgery. I had one of those awful visions of impending disaster – dog biting owner, dog biting nurse, dog having horrendous anaesthetic reaction, me dropping an ovarian stump and searching frantically through a blood-filled abdomen with owner sobbing brokenly in the corner ... None of those things happened, thank the lord, but the strain was intense.

I'm feeling a little bit seedy. While idly pondering the potential causes, I realised that today I have eaten:

- Two pieces of white toast with butter and marmalade
- Two pieces of Black Forest gateau
- Two slices of pizza
- One mini Twix bar
- Five cups of coffee
- A large glass of red wine
- A bowl of macaroni cheese

Not really a shining example of a healthy, balanced diet. I did take an apple to work with me, but since I brought it home again and put it back into the fruit bowl, I don't think I can count it.

Wednesday 8 July

Wet, cold day. Blake spent last night at a friend's house, and when I picked him up at four, he came staggering out of the lounge, dazed and blinking, having spent twenty-four hours playing *Minecraft*. He explained all the way home how important it is that we get *Minecraft* too, so he can play at home. Over my dead body.

In the evening I went out to our annual practice-wide educational evening, where every vet and technician has to give a five-minute talk. It used to go on for *hours*, but a couple of years ago Grant the sales rep was appointed timekeeper, and his policy of an alarm at four and a half minutes and shouting, 'Shut up and sit down! You've had your time!' at five minutes has kept things crisp and snappy ever since.

    We all complain bitterly about the educational evening, but it's actually really good fun. It's nice to catch up with everyone, and we get Thai for dinner as a bribe. I talked about doing cow abdominal surgery with the patient on her back rather than on her feet as described by the textbooks – it's much easier to reach the bits you need to. Someone gave an excellent talk about how to remove a retained placenta from a mare – I'm still not at all keen to do it myself, but I'm delighted to learn that the expert is only an hour away. Someone else talked about Varroa mites and deformed wing virus in a beehive – fascinating – and there was a great presentation on a case of yew-tree poisoning in cattle, with 30 seconds spent on the poisoning and four and a half minutes of interesting yew-tree-related trivia and photos of his recent overseas trip.

Thursday 9 July

I've been trying to organise visits to and from kids' friends during the holidays. It's making my head hurt. Both children have best friends, good friends and friends that will do if nobody else is available. So, of course, do the friends, and the rankings aren't necessarily the same from both directions.

Ellie's best friend is child A1 (family A, oldest child). Her *second*-best friend is B1, who is best friends with A2. Blake is good friends with B2 but better friends with C2. C1 is best friends with B2. Then there's family D – Blake's best friend is D2 (although I think that D2's favourite friend is actually someone completely different), but Ellie and D1 don't get on at all. Both B1 and B2 are good friends with D3. Every family has various prior commitments, and every parent's work schedule is different. Even if we sent around a group spreadsheet, we'd never be able to make every child happy.

Anyway, the current plan is for Ellie to spend two nights next week at the A's place, and then one night with family B. B2 will come to our place – unless the C's are back from their grandparents' place, in which case B2 and C1 will hang out, and C2 will spend the night with us.

Friday 10 July

An excellent day. The sun shone, I spent a couple of happy hours this morning filling bait stations and some even happier hours this afternoon constructing my new brick path. (Path construction went even better once I'd removed the pissed-off earwig from inside my left gardening glove. Ugghhh.) The kids went over to Sean and Amy's and returned with their three little girls, who were all very keen on path construction. They spent a happy half-hour digging holes in my pile of crusher dust before they all started bickering and telling on each other, and I sent the little girls home again, with Blake as escort to make sure nobody fell in a swamp on the way.

We watched *9 to 5* after dinner, on the grounds that anything involving Dolly Parton was guaranteed to be fabulous. It was.

Monday 13 July

Today I received a scrotum. As one does. It belonged to a bull I saw last week that had a raging temperature and one big testicle. I put him on antibiotics and anti-inflammatories, but he died on Saturday. The farmer texted to let me know, and I asked him if we could send some tissue off to the lab. I've never seen a testicular infection in a bull, but according to the textbooks there are various nasty venereal diseases, all exotic to New Zealand, that could cause such a thing.

The scrotum arrived in a chilly bag, surrounded by ice bricks. I cut it open, and found a nasty-looking bruise on the testicle and a whole lot of foul-smelling pus heading up the spermatic cord. Diagnosis: a kick to the groin resulting in a haematoma, which then got infected. (In cattle, haematomas quite often do turn into abscesses.) The infection probably tracked all the way up into the abdomen, and death was most likely due to peritonitis. A horrible thing to happen, but not, thank goodness, the first national case of some hideous exotic disease.

I was returning the scrotum to the plastic bag it came in to throw it away when I noticed that, either by design or happy accident, the farmer had sent it in an old Yellow Pages bag, with MAY CONTAIN NUTS printed across it in large capital letters. Totally made my day.

It's time to bring this diary to an end. Past time – my year was up two days ago. I was planning to finish with an uplifting and inspirational paragraph about the simple, wholesome joys of country life. But on second thoughts, that's a little trite. Ending a book with an infected scrotum, on the other hand, has probably never been done before.

Epilogue

Clare sold her small-animal practice six months after moving in with Dan. She has taken to dairy farming like a duck to water, transformed Dan's calf sheds from perfectly adequate to totally amazing, and is steadfastly refusing all job offers from local vet clinics. She and Dan are very happy; these days, he always smiles and waves when you pass him on the road.

Sophie is now the creator and star of the smash-hit Netflix show *Here's One I Spayed Earlier*, in which she demonstrates veterinary procedures with her trademark poise and infectious giggle. After declaring that she's far too busy being an influencer to think about boys, she has just embarked on a whirlwind love affair with her producer.

Val and Trevor went to Nelson for the weekend, and announced on their return that they'd got married while they were away. This caused a certain amount of outrage from both their families, which they serenely ignored. Val says she always wanted to elope, and it was just as much fun as she'd hoped.

Ellie is enjoying boarding school, despite grave concerns that her family are incapable of properly looking after the pigs, dogs, cat, pet rams and goat in her absence.

Blake plans to be an All Black, a professional free-runner and a trick cyclist when he grows up. His preferred training method is to watch videos on YouTube, and he greets with amused scorn suggestions that actually practising is the best way to improve.

The timber for James's new cattle yards arrived last week, the heifers are growing well and the ewes are set-stocked for lambing in plenty of grass. He is a happy man.

The back door handle has still not been fixed, which is disappointing. But the bathroom light has, and the new brick path is a symphony of practicality and style.

And Danielle, whose latest international bestseller was described by the *New York Times* as 'warm, witty, fresh, charming, breathtaking in scope and altogether delightful' and by her sister-in-law as 'can't see what all the fuss is about, to be honest', has managed to remain unaffected by fame and fortune. She still works part-time as a vet, and spends her enormous royalty cheques on predator-proof fences and large-scale wetland restoration projects. (Alright, I made that up. But it's fun to dream.)

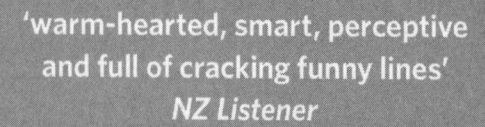

'warm-hearted, smart, perceptive and full of cracking funny lines'
NZ Listener

Danielle Hawkins

the pretty delicious café

One flaky family.
One ex-boyfriend who won't go away.
And one handsome stranger who probably will ...

THE PRETTY DELICIOUS CAFÉ

One flaky family. One ex-boyfriend who won't go away. And one handsome stranger who probably will ... For fans of *Doc Martin* and Monica McInerney, a warm, witty novel, brimming with the trademark romance, friendship and eccentricity that Danielle Hawkins's readers love.

On the outskirts of a small seaside town, Lia and her friend Anna work serious hours running their restored café. The summer season is upon them, they have Anna's wedding to plan and Lia's ex-boyfriend seems not to understand it's over.

When a gorgeous stranger taps on Lia's window near midnight and turns out not to be a serial killer, she feels it's a promising sign. But no one comes without a past, and his arrives in the form of a four-year-old son. Just as Lia decides to give things a try, problems from her own past rear up.

The Pretty Delicious Café reminds us of the joy – and hazards – to be found in family, friends and good food – and that being a little bit weird isn't necessarily a bad thing.

'At last a single mum as heroine! A romantic tale capturing the all too realistic challenges of single parenthood with humour and hope. I didn't want it to end.' Jacinta Tynan

when it all went to custard

Odds of saving marriage – slim.
Farming expertise – patchy.
Chances that it'll all be okay in the end
– actually pretty good.

Danielle Hawkins

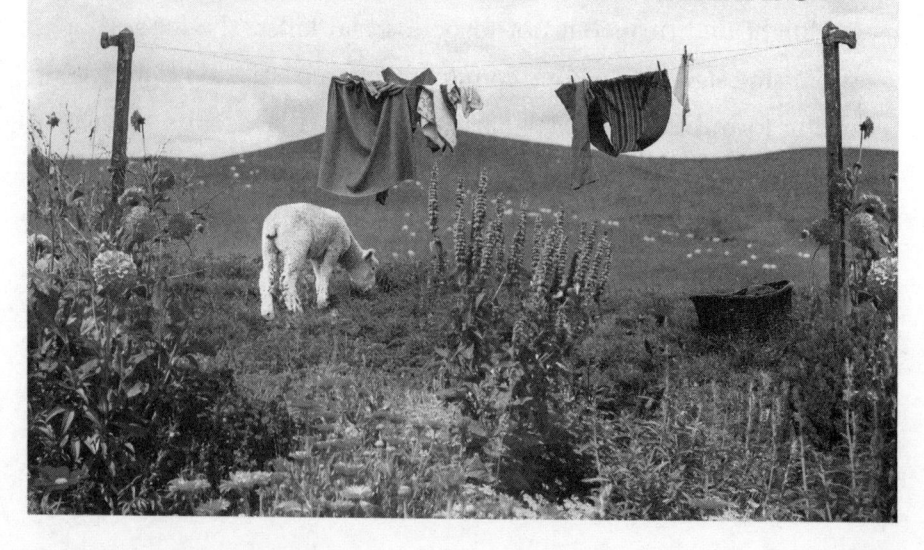

WHEN IT ALL WENT TO CUSTARD

Odds of saving marriage – slim. Farming expertise – patchy. Chances that it'll all be okay in the end – actually pretty good ...

For those who love *Eleanor Oliphant is Completely Fine*, Alexander McCall Smith and novels with heart, soul and a dose of common sense.

> *I wasn't enjoying the afternoon of 23 February even before I learnt that my husband was having an affair ...*

The news of her husband's infidelity comes as a nasty shock to Jenny Reynolds, part-time building control officer and full-time mother – even though, to her surprise and embarrassment, her first reaction is relief, not anguish. What really hurts is her children's unhappiness at the break-up, and the growing realisation that, alone, she may lose the family farm.

This is the story of the year after Jenny's old life falls apart; of family and farming, pet lambs and geriatric dogs, choko-bearing tenants and Springsteen-esque neighbours. And of just perhaps a second chance at happiness.